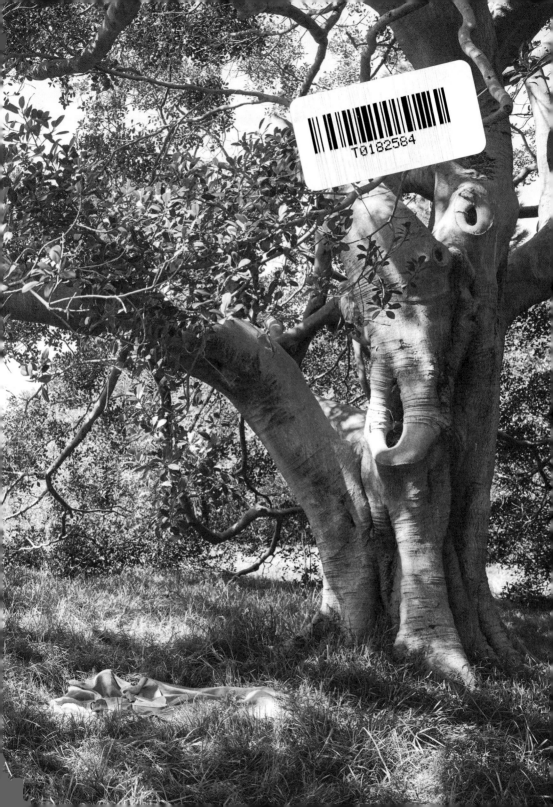

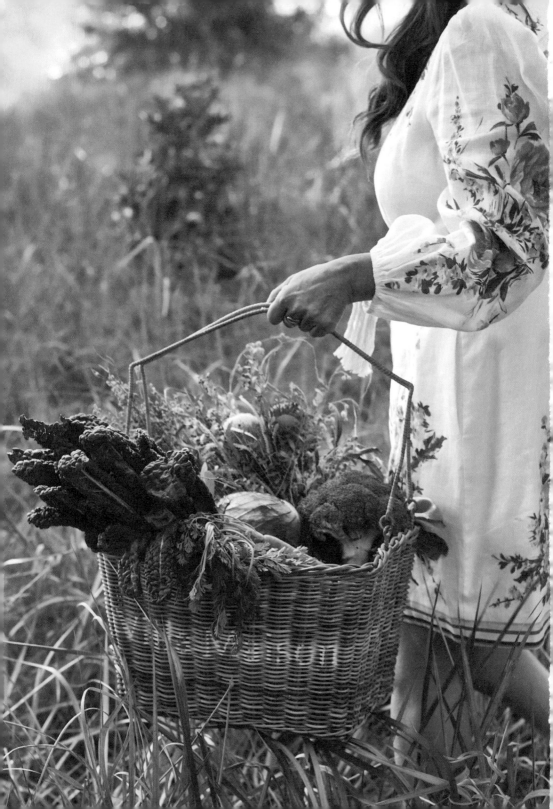

About the author

Meet Lee Holmes, the force behind all things supercharged. She's a qualified clinical nutritionist, yoga and meditation teacher, wholefoods chef and author of the bestselling *Supercharged Food* series. Her 10 books include *Eat Yourself Beautiful*, *Heal Your Gut* and the page-turner *Supercharge Your Life*.

When she's not whipping up gut-friendly concoctions in her kitchen, you'll find Lee running her successful online health programs, 'Heal Your Gut' and 'Fast Your Way to Wellness'. She's a regular columnist for *Wellbeing* and *Eat Well* magazines, and a regular on ABC Radio in Australia. Lee's articles have been published across the globe in prestigious publications like *The Times*, *The Telegraph*, *The Guardian*, *The Daily Express* and *The Australian*.

Lee's website, superchargeyourgut.com, is a gut health haven offering powders and blends including the popular Love Your Gut powder. And her award-winning cooking blog, superchargedfood.com, is a treasure trove of SOLE food: sustainable, organic, local and ethical. You'll find drool-worthy recipes, tantalising information, nutrition news, product reviews and menu-planning ideas that will make your tastebuds tingle.

Contact Lee at lee@superchargedfood.com
Follow her adventures at

- /superchargedfood
- /LeeSupercharged
- /leesupercharged
- /leeholmes67
- /leesupercharged

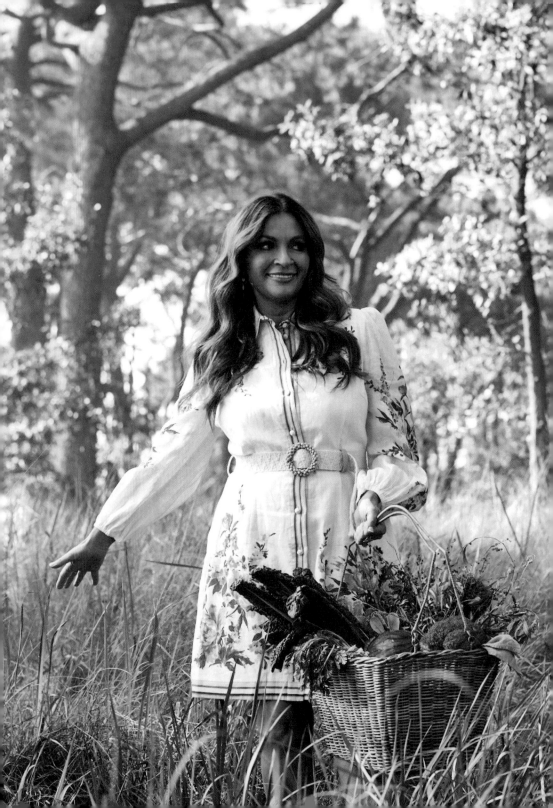

Lee Holmes

Nature's Way to Healing

A Long Covid guide

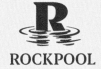

ROCKPOOL

A Rockpool book

PO Box 252

Summer Hill

NSW 2130

Australia

rockpoolpublishing.com

Follow us! **f** **⊙** rockpoolpublishing

Tag your images with #rockpoolpublishing

ISBN: 9781922786043

Published in 2024 by Rockpool Publishing

Styling: Vanessa Austin, vanessaaustin.com

Food preparation: Miche Bloch and Emma Norton

Make-up: Louise Antonjik, louiseantonjuk.com

Images pp. 18, 43, 54, 74, 79, 98, 106, 109, 185,
236 & 241: Unsplash; p. 46: Lee Holmes

Design and typesetting by Christine Armstrong, Rockpool Publishing

Edited by Jess Cox

A catalogue record for this
book is available from the
National Library of Australia

NATIONAL
LIBRARY
OF AUSTRALIA

Printed and bound in China

10 9 8 7 6 5 4 3 2 1

Contents

Dinner

Snacks

Other

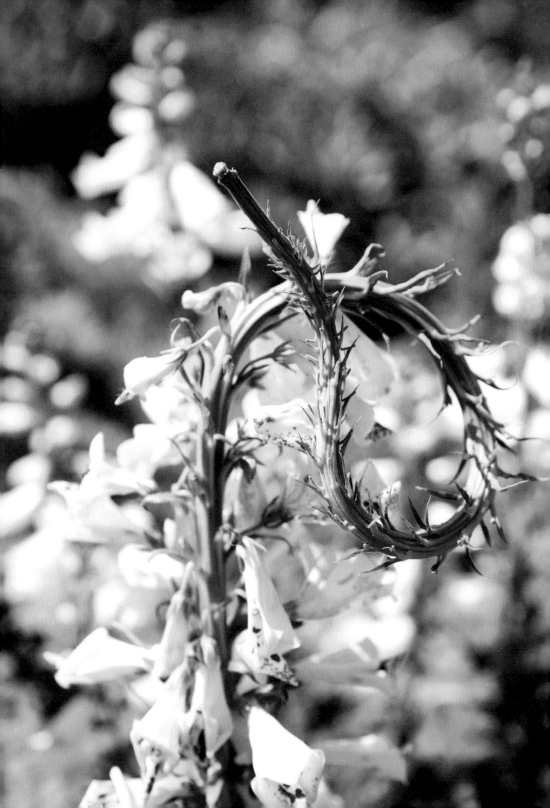

List of abbreviations

ACE2	Angiotensin-converting enzyme 2
ANS	Autonomic nervous system
ATP	Adenosine triphosphate
CBD	Cannabidiol
CFS	Chronic fatigue syndrome
CNS	Central nervous system
CRP	C-reactive protein
DAO	Diamine oxidase
DVT	Deep vein thrombosis
EBV	Epstein–Barr virus
GERD	Gastro-oesophageal reflux disease
GP	General practitioner
IL-6	Interleukin-6
IVIG	Intravenous immunoglobulin
LDN	Low-dose naltrexone
MCAS	Mast cell activation syndrome
ME	Myalgic encephalomyelitis
NAC	N-acetylcysteine
PAIS	Post-infectious autoimmune syndrome
PASC	Post-acute sequelae of SARS-CoV-2 infection
PE	Pulmonary embolism
PEM	Post-exertional malaise
PNS	Peripheral nervous system
POTS	Postural orthostatic tachycardia syndrome
PTSD	Post-traumatic stress disorder
RAT	Rapid antigen test
REM	Rapid eye movement
RNA	Ribonucleic acid
SNS	Sympathetic nervous system
UK	United Kingdom
USA	United States of America

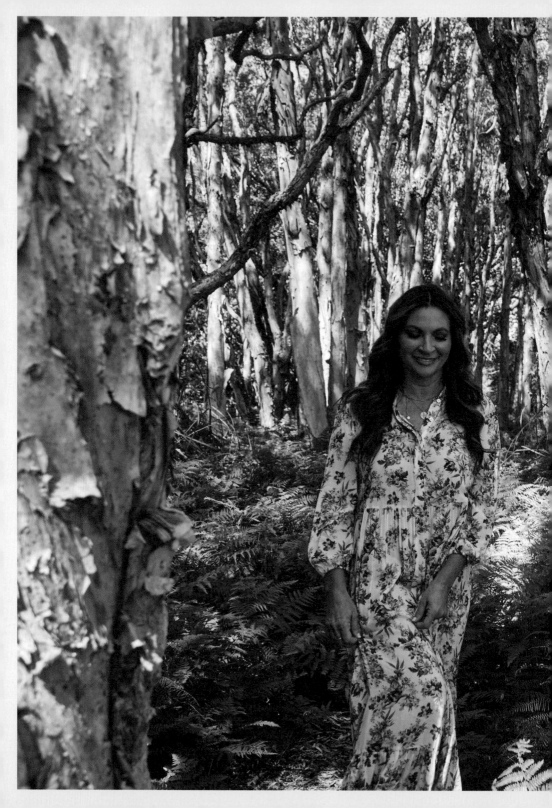

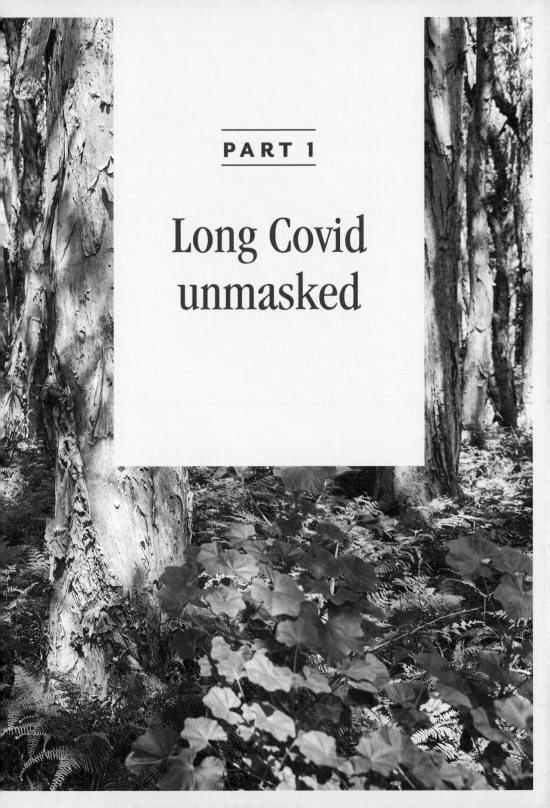

PART 1

Long Covid
unmasked

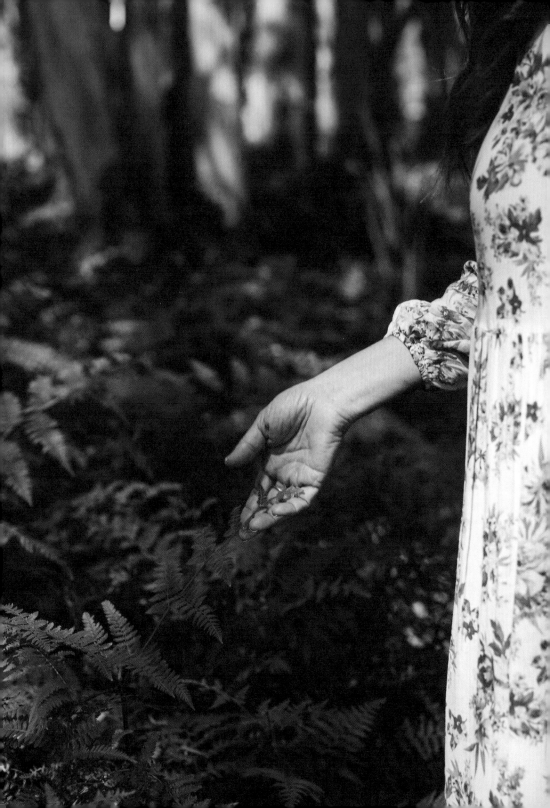

Ah, the C-word.
No, not that C-word!
The other one.
Covid.

The C-word

It's been more than three years since we first heard about the dreaded C-word. While it turned our world upside down for a period of time, for some, it feels as though the dust has settled and Covid has become a distant memory.

For others, however, COVID-19 has had a longer-term impact, whether it's because they've lost a loved one or because of its mental and physical toll. Being treated in a hospital emergency room or intensive care for Covid has even resulted in post-traumatic stress disorder (PTSD).[1]

When it comes to Long Covid, I'm right here with you. It's hard to fathom that, in some parts of the world, Long Covid affects one in five people. In the United States of America (USA) alone, more than 49 million people are currently living with Long Covid. Worldwide, sufferers are estimated in the realms of 100 million.[2]

If you've had Covid, you'll have almost a 50 per cent chance of going on to experience Long Covid. Women make up a disproportionate share of Long Covid patients. Affectionately known as 'long-haulers', these brave individuals have my upmost admiration. These selfless souls are the canaries in a coal mine, and their experiences are providing great insights into post-viral

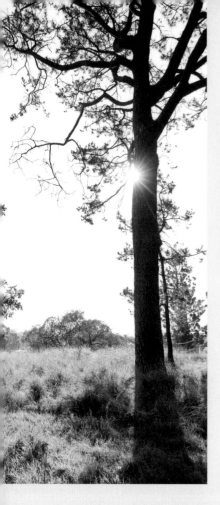

illness, immune system dysregulation and a fractured medical system, as well as empathy and human connection.

I've written this book specifically for my fellow long-haulers, because I want to give you the tools you need to recover more quickly and get back to enjoying life. Forget random, costly and unresearched solutions – here is a practical, day-by-day and up-to-the-minute plan that is tried and tested and has long-term positive results.

As a qualified clinical nutritionist, I've developed a protocol that works. Evidence is still being uncovered and can take years to develop, and I didn't have years to spare, especially because my life's purpose is to help others with their health and wellness. With so many millions of people impaired, we have an urgent need for accelerating clinical trials with promising immune system–modulating or virus-inactivating agents. So with the help of my own research and input from specialised medical doctors at the forefront of emerging Long Covid research globally, I've created a holistic approach to Long Covid that will not only help to improve symptoms but also get to their root cause.

This book includes a nutritional protocol and support plan, delicious simple-to-make recipes, an easy-to-follow menu plan and list of low-histamine foods. I've compiled resources to make it easier for you too; you can document your progress with a Monthly Symptom Tracker, self-evaluate and record your improvements and manage your self-care and recovery through a Weekly Self-care Checklist and Pacing Diary. I've got your back every step of the way, because I know firsthand how debilitating Long Covid can be. Together we've got this.

My Long Covid journey

I picked up COVID-19 on a trip to the United Kingdom (UK) and was diagnosed in late spring 2022 after experiencing clusters and constellations of symptoms that emerged then dissipated. They came in waves, cropping up at regular intervals just when I thought I was approaching the finishing line.

When I did the rapid antigen test (RAT), the positive pink line felt like more an inconvenience than anything else. I was due to fly back to Sydney in a week and didn't welcome the self-enforced isolation. Being exiled from family and friends was not something I was pleased about. I had already been away for three months and was itching to get back home. Every cell in my body wanted to flee. I was yearning to feel the warmth of the sun on my skin among the frangipani-lined Northern Beaches, bobbing along in my old-school Nordic boat, safely cocooned in the gentle waves of Pittwater. I pictured myself working at my desk, with my cheeky cat Tinkerbell sprawled on top of my computer, supervising, while in the background, the cicadas' orchestral sounds filled the air.

The first COVID-19 symptoms felt almost flu-like: generalised fatigue; a pinchy, throbbing headache; fevers that left the bedsheets drenched; and irrational chills that would come and go. I'd fling off the bedspread during the rapid flames that engulfed my body, then cling to it as teeth-chattering shivers took hold, muscles tightening and relaxing in rapid succession.

I spent my nights meandering between sleep and wakefulness, thoughts flicking and hovering between endurance and positivity. After a few days, I started to notice my symptoms were shapeshifting: feather-like one minute, offering a beacon of hope, then hitting me smack bang over the head with a sledgehammer, sending me straight back to square one.

With hopes fading fast, I was held captive, with a heavy aching chest pain that felt like my heart was exploding out of my chest. It worsened and developed into post-exertion chest pain. Struggling for breath, I felt imprisoned. Whenever I tried to exert myself – even when attempting a slow walk around the block – I became stationary, hunched over and trapped in a physical and mental flight-or-fight response. It was exhausting.

Nothing seemed to work. The unrelenting fatigue was crippling, the brain fog intoxicating and my old life had become a far distant memory, overtaken by a fuddled brain and confusion. The rich colour of the outside world was fading; the walls were closing in. I felt weary, consumed with my inner life and the gloomy muddled way I was feeling. It was starting to break me down. Merciless hours turned into days then weeks lying in bed, unable to see the light at the end of the tunnel. My possibilities narrowed; moment by moment, my health began to slip away. As this new harsh reality settled in, I found myself unable to work and interact with the world around me, unable to cope with even the simplest of tasks. I was overwhelmed by a world that seemed increasingly large and frightening. All I wanted to do was curl up in a foetal position and sleep.

The weather in the UK was turning from summer to autumn. Days were shortening, the air felt crisper as it whistled through a small crack above the flaky window ledge and brittle leaves were beginning to collect in piles around the entrance door. It was almost a month later when this soon to be long-hauler hauled my aching body out of bed and took a long-haul flight back to the Land of Oz, touching down with both joy and elation, but trepidation at the thought of crawling up 46 stairs to get to my front door. As I sat at the bottom of the staircase with barely any energy to spare, I knew I had to start crawling up. The climb felt insurmountable.

Post-exertional malaise (PEM) had started to affect my day-to-day life, and I knew that once inside, I would need to rest for days to recover from the exertion of the trip home. If I didn't, I had learned by now that the palpitations, fatigue, brain fog, dizziness and malaise would soon return in full force.

After experiencing COVID-19, I noticed that my previous run-in with chronic fatigue syndrome (CFS), also known as myalgic encephalomyelitis (ME), which I'd had in my 20s, had now re-emerged and my mast cell activation syndrome (MCAS) reactivated. I was in the middle of a tiring relapse. My mast cells (the immune-cell ringleaders in the immune response) were fuming; my skin was alive with hives; even the thin air around me felt heavy and prickly. My immune system had gone haywire and was misbehaving like a petulant child. Heart palpitations and tachycardia ensued; inflammation decided to run amok throughout my body. I immediately sought medical help. I was diagnosed with post-viral illness and pericarditis (inflammation around the pericardium of the heart). While I have always aimed to be big-hearted, I think Covid took this a bit literally!

Keen to access specialist care and not attempt to self-diagnose or self-treat these unusual symptoms, I sought out medical intervention. On my way to the cardiologist, the short walk sent my heart rate up to 160 beats per minute; orthostatic intolerance had set in and another post-exertion crash (or payback) was imminent, which would see me couchbound for days.

So here I was – a natural health practitioner, the author of 10 books about nutritional health and an expert in my field and a healthy, active, vibrant person – now part of the Long Covid 'lived experience' and barely able to muster the energy to seek help for myself.

I left the cardiologist clutching a prescription for colchicine, an anti-inflammatory medication prescribed for pericarditis, with the same ache in my heart. I felt defeated, disillusioned and confused. My specialist had been seeing patients with Long Covid day in and day out. Many looked normal from the outside, and he admitted to feeling perplexed and saddened by his lack of answers. He went home each night worrying about his patients and feeling inadequate, unable to provide the answers they so desperately needed.

While Long Covid sounds like a recent phenomenon, it's been impacting people's lives globally for a few years now, and long-haulers are looking for answers. Unfortunately, the pace of research is sluggish. The medical system doesn't have the answers or resources to care for Long Covid patients. People who aren't in a medical field may visit their primary care doctor, such as a general practitioner (GP), who will decide whether further examination or specialty care is necessary.

Given how slowly research is unfolding, GPs don't always have the answers and recommend for patients to access further treatment. Some doctors don't believe Long Covid is a real condition and medical gaslighting can ensue, even at a subtle level. It's not always easy to spot, but some signs are that your healthcare provider doesn't seem to be an engaged listener and continually interrupts you while you're talking. They may minimise or downplay what you're experiencing, or you may feel like your provider is rude, condescending or demeaning towards you. If this happens to you, remember that you are the expert on your own body. It's important to tune in to your body and advocate for yourself.

If you find yourself in this position, consider writing down detailed notes and records of your symptoms. You can opt to bring a support person with you to your next appointment, or even look for a new healthcare provider.

Once my appointment was over, I trundled down the steps, into the open air, and I remember a multitude of questions rattling around in my head: 'How did I get pericarditis?' 'Why has my chronic fatigue and MCAS flared up?' 'Is there a connection?' 'Why is this happening to me?' 'Am I cursed?'

During my subsequent science-nerd researching to answer these questions, I had an epiphany about Long Covid and its potential links to mast cell activation and dysregulated immune response. I studiously typed this subject into the PubMed website. To my astonishment, the latest research corroborated my gut instincts. There was a connection between the two – they were taking centre stage in the latest research studies.

I discovered that Long Covid's resemblance to other chronic ailments such as ME/CFS was finally providing insight into its causes and treatments, and spearheading even more studies. I knew then I was on to something. I was keen to learn as much as I could, but I also needed to pace myself and rest, because as a long-hauler myself, I was well aware that pushing through can harm the recovery and healing process. I didn't want to miss anything along the way or have details become translucent over time. So I decided to put pen to paper. During the process of experiencing and learning, I began documenting everything.

Each step forward is a stride
towards wellness. Trust your steady
inner compass; it will help you
navigate this current storm.

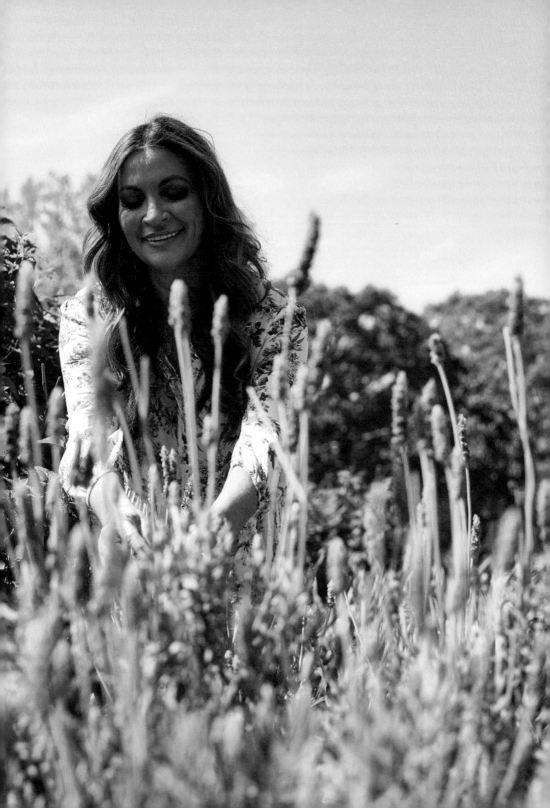

Long Covid is an intricate tapestry of multiple systems and symptoms, repetitively hamster-wheeling though your system.

The science behind Long Covid

They say patience is a virtue, but with Long Covid, it's more like a job requirement. Have you ever seen the movie *Groundhog Day*? For the main character, every day is the same. With Long Covid, it's living the same day over and over again, but being hit with even more fatigue, brain fog and shortness of breath as the days roll on. The brain fog makes you forget much of your day before, until a few months down the track when you slowly come out of it. Reality sets in and you realise you're living through *Groundhog Day*. You relive the same hamster-wheeling day, but with a cloudy mind so you can't even enjoy the small pleasures that come with repetition, like knowing the good bits or having a semblance of a routine. No, you basically stumble through your day, trying to remember what you did yesterday, but all you can recall is a vague sense of déjà vu. It's only when scratching your head that you realise you haven't washed your hair in days. When you're stuck in *Groundhog Day* with brain fog, all you can really do is laugh – or cry. Preferably laugh. Because the good news is that this is temporary and you will get through it.

Long Covid is a complex and often debilitating condition that can affect individuals who have recovered from an initial SARS-CoV-2 infection. While the exact cause of Long Covid is still being studied, it is related to the body's immune response to the virus. In some cases, it may have a neurological and thrombotic, cardiovascular component.

In May 2020, Elisa Perego, from the Institute of Archaeology at University College London,[3] first used the term #LongCovid on Twitter to describe her personal experience with the condition. While Long Covid has become a widely recognised term, other phrases are also used, such as post-acute sequelae of SARS-CoV-2 infection (PASC), post-COVID-19, post-acute COVID-19 syndrome, chronic Covid syndrome and chronic COVID-19.

Long Covid is generally described as when people's health hasn't returned to their prior health after having COVID-19. The World Health Organization reports, 'Long Covid is defined as lasting for three months from infection, lasts at least two months, and can't be explained by another diagnosis.'[4]

Each case of COVID-19 is unique; each person has a different experience in their recovery. People can start to feel better, then get a flare-up of symptoms after experiencing something stressful or getting sick and take a few months to get better.

Patients with Long Covid report prolonged, multisystem involvement and significant disability. Seven months later, many patients are not yet recovered (mainly from systemic and neurological/cognitive symptoms), have not returned to their previous levels of work and continue to experience significant symptoms.[5]

To grasp the concept of Long Covid, we need to understand how SARS-CoV-2 infects the body. The virus enters the cells by binding to the angiotensin-converting enzyme 2 (ACE2) receptor. This attachment triggers an increase in angiotensin levels, which leads to inflammation, vasoconstriction and thrombosis. SARS-CoV-2 also needs a protease to prime the spike protein before entering the cell. The ACE2 receptor and protease are found in various parts of the body, including the lungs, heart, smooth muscle in the gut, liver, kidney, neurons and immune cells.

Severe Long Covid symptoms may result from reduced ACE2 activity, even in people who did not get sick. This decline can interfere with energy metabolism and mitochondria (the organelles inside cells that produce energy) and lead to issues such as cardiac problems, pneumonia, blood clots, kidney failure, strokes, seizures, brain fog, excessive inflammation and autoimmune disease.

Long Covid may affect how the mitochondria functions; mitochondria provide energy to our cells and metabolism, which is particularly important for organs that require a lot of energy such as the brain, heart and muscles. COVID-19 can damage the mitochondria in various organs, leading to decreased energy production and increased oxidative stress. This may contribute to some symptoms of Long Covid such as fatigue, brain fog and muscle weakness.

Because the gastrointestinal tract has many ACE2 receptors, COVID-19 can disrupt the balance of bacteria in the gut, leading to gut dysbiosis and inflammation. Long Covid is not limited to individuals who had COVID-19; it is also being observed in some people who have received COVID-19 vaccines, possibly due to autoantibodies targeting the ACE2 receptor, which the spike protein targets.

Long Covid may be associated with changes in gene expression and cellular metabolism. For example, a study published in *Nature* found that individuals with Long Covid had alterations in the genes involved in inflammation, metabolism and mitochondrial function, among others.[7] Another study found that Long Covid patients had differences in the metabolism of immune cells called T cells, which could contribute to ongoing immune dysregulation.[8]

According to a recent study in *Scientific American,*[9] Long Covid may actually be a neurological disease, which could explain the wide range of symptoms patients experience. Many individuals with Long Covid had neurological symptoms, including confusion, memory problems and even seizures. The findings suggest that doctors should focus on treating the neurological symptoms of Long Covid, as well as managing other symptoms such as fatigue and pain.

New research published in *Science Advances*[10] indicates that COVID-19 can cause brain cells to fuse, potentially leading to long-term neurological symptoms such as brain fog, headaches and loss of taste and smell. This fusion may enable the virus to evade the immune system, which could explain its presence in the brains of Long Covid patients even months after infection. The study sheds light on the possible mechanism behind chronic neurological symptoms in COVID patients.

Many individuals with Long Covid experience cognitive dysfunction, such as difficulty with memory, attention, sleep and mood, which are easily recognised as brain or nerve related. Other symptoms seem to be more physical than neurological, such as pain and PEM, a type of 'energy crash' that occurs even after mild exercise. These symptoms are also due to nerve dysfunction, particularly in the autonomic nervous system, which regulates our bodily functions such as breathing and digestion. Known as dysautonomia, this condition can lead to dizziness, rapid heartbeat, high or low blood pressure and gastrointestinal issues, often leaving individuals unable to work or function independently.

'I now think of COVID as a neurological disease as much as I think of it as a pulmonary disease, and that's definitely true in Long Covid,' says William Pittman, a physician at UCLA Health in Los Angeles, USA. By identifying Long Covid as partly a neurological disease, doctors can now focus on treating the root cause of this condition, rather than simply managing the symptoms.

What causes Long Covid?

Long Covid can develop in young, healthy individuals following a mild initial infection of COVID-19, but the risk of developing this condition is slightly higher in older adults and those who were hospitalised for COVID-19. Women and individuals facing socioeconomic disadvantage are also at higher risk, as are those who smoke, are obese or have pre-existing health conditions, particularly autoimmune diseases. In 2021, a meta-analysis of 41 studies revealed that, worldwide, 43 per cent of individuals infected with SARS-CoV-2 may develop Long Covid.[11]

The exact cause and underlying mechanisms of Long Covid are still not fully understood, but they are related to how the virus affects the body's immune system and organ function. Theories include persistent viral

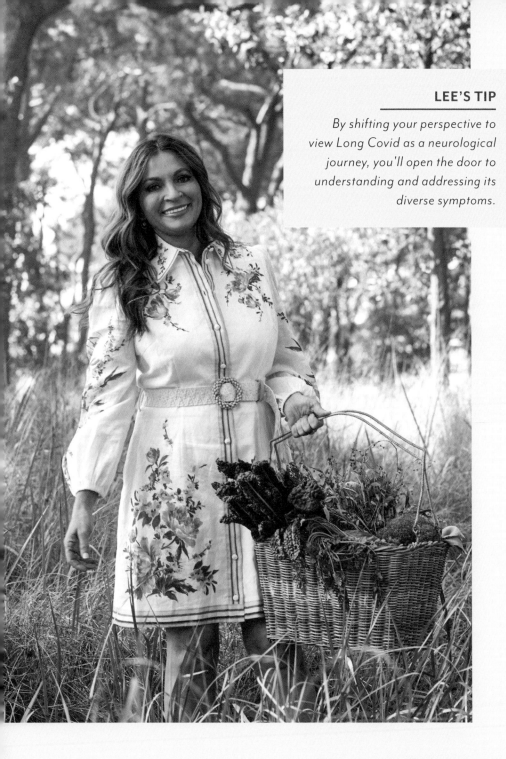

LEE'S TIP

By shifting your perspective to view Long Covid as a neurological journey, you'll open the door to understanding and addressing its diverse symptoms.

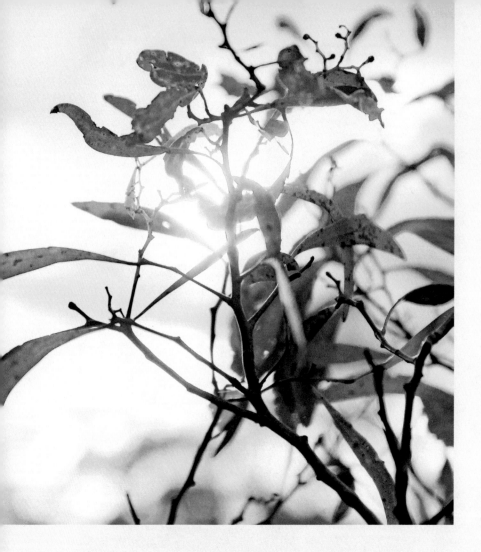

infection, reactivation of a latent virus or the presence of inactivated viral fragments. Some scientists speculate that an immune response triggered by pro-inflammatory cytokines may be involved.

Studies have shown that COVID-19 can induce systemic inflammation,[12] which in turn can lead to an increase in pro-inflammatory cytokines and adaptive immunity (specialised cells that eliminate pathogens). This mechanism is thought to play a critical role in regulating the immune system. There are 10 main potential factors and mechanisms that may contribute to the development and persistence of Long Covid symptoms.

10 POTENTIAL FACTORS AND MECHANISMS FOR LONG COVID	
Viral persistence	The SARS-CoV-2 virus can persist in some individuals, causing ongoing inflammation and damage to tissues and organs. Viral ribonucleic acid (RNA) can be found in various body parts even months after initial infection.
Immune system dysfunction	Disruptions in the immune system's response to COVID-19 can lead to ongoing inflammation and tissue damage, resulting from a persistent autoimmune response or overactive immune function.
Mast cell activation	Activated mast cells release substances that trigger an immune response, causing symptoms such as itching and swelling. Hyperinflammation from this activation may contribute to Long Covid symptoms.
Reactivation of dormant viruses	COVID-19 can reactivate dormant viruses in the body, causing health issues.
Chronic fatigue recurrence	Long Covid symptoms overlap with post-acute infection and chronic fatigue syndromes, suggesting a common underlying cause.
Autophagy dysregulation	Autophagy refers to the cleaning up and reusing of damaged cell parts. If this process is dysregulated, it may hinder the immune system's ability to clear the virus, leading to viral persistence and prolonged symptoms. It can also contribute to tissue damage and inflammation.
Endothelial dysfunction	COVID-19 can cause dysfunction in the endothelium (the lining of blood vessels), leading to blood clots and organ damage.
Neurological damage	The virus can cause inflammation and injury to the brain and nervous system, resulting in neurological symptoms.
Damage to organs	COVID-19 can damage various organs, and post-inflammatory responses may contribute to Long Covid symptoms.
Mental health factors	The stress and trauma of the pandemic and COVID-19 infection may contribute to ongoing mental health symptoms.

These mechanisms are not mutually exclusive; they may interact with one another to contribute to Long Covid.

✴ UNDERSTANDING THE 'SPIKE PROTEIN' ✴

Before I had Covid, the thought of a spike protein was as alien to me as finding toilet paper in a grocery store in the middle of a pandemic. If someone had told me five years ago that I'd spend months researching it, I'd have laughed my ACE2 off!

The spike protein is a key feature of the SARS-CoV-2 virus, which causes COVID-19. It protrudes from the virus's surface and helps the virus bind to and enter human cells. The spike protein binds to a specific receptor called the ACE2 receptor. Once attached to the ACE2 receptor, the virus can enter the human cell and begin to replicate itself.

The spike protein is also the primary target of COVID-19 vaccines, which work by giving the body the genetic instructions to produce the spike protein, thus teaching the immune system to recognise and produce antibodies against it. Vaccinated people have been shown to develop Long Covid symptoms.

The spike protein may play a role in Long Covid.[13] Its presence in the body, even after the virus has been cleared, can trigger an immune response leading to inflammation of and damage to various organs and tissues. It can bind to ACE2 receptors on cells throughout the body,[14] not just the respiratory tract, allowing the virus to enter and infect cells in other organs such as the heart, brain, kidneys and gastrointestinal tract.

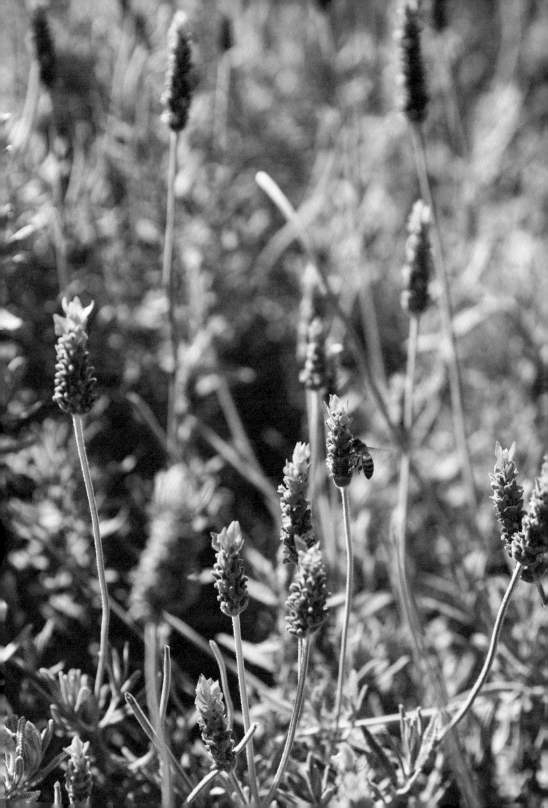

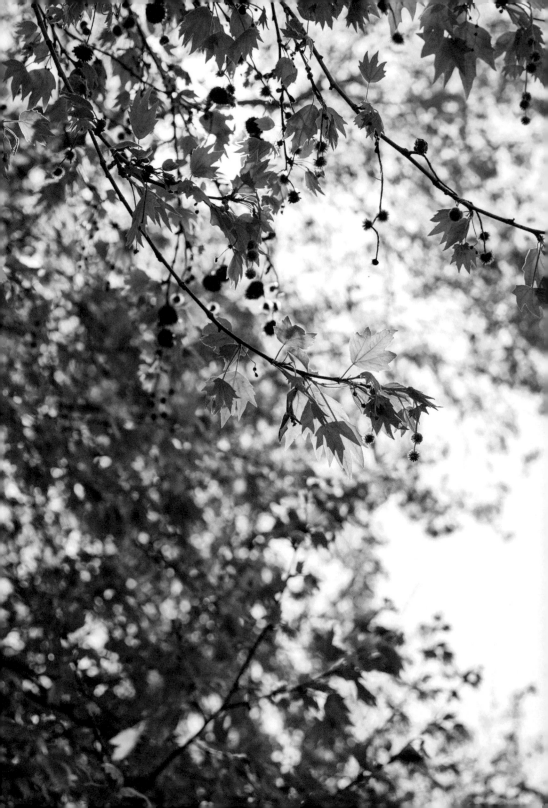

Your feelings are the road map to healing. Every sensation is a signpost guiding you forward.

Is what I'm feeling Long Covid?

Common symptoms

Maybe you're reading this book because you've been diagnosed with Long Covid, or you know someone who has. Or maybe you're feeling achy and brain foggy, and wonder why you haven't bounced back from COVID-19 like your friends or family have. It can be scary when you're not sure what's going on with your body and it's not performing as it should, no matter what you do. It's like a giant game of Cluedo, except that instead of Colonel Mustard in the library with a candlestick, it's you and millions of others taking wild guesses in a darkened conservatory.

Let's face it: with the fatigue, pins and needles and achiness you might have found yourself scouring the internet for compression stockings, or wondering whether these strange bodily sensations are just because you're getting older. Before you start planning your retirement, let's explore the different symptoms of Long Covid to see what resonates with you. Maybe you can finally put a name to the weird phenomena you've been feeling and understand why it's happening? And you'll have a good excuse for forgetting things and needing that extra afternoon nap when people are tut-tutting at you, thinking you're being lazy!

In the chapters ahead, we'll look at how you can shorten Long Covid's lifespan and improve your symptoms.

Symptoms of Long Covid

Long Covid has more than 200 potential symptoms spread across 10 different organ systems, which you could experience in different stages of the disease. Symptoms include fatigue, brain fog, shortness of breath, cognitive dysfunction, chest pain, joint pain, headaches, loss of smell or taste, difficulty sleeping and an impact on everyday functioning. Some people with Long Covid may also experience depression, anxiety or other mental health problems. Symptoms of Long Covid may either emerge as new onset following the initial recovery from acute COVID-19 or persist from the illness. They may fluctuate or relapse over time.

The following diagram shows commonly reported Long Covid symptoms. Are you suffering from any of them? Circle each one that affects you, and notice how many you are experiencing and what areas of the body they are in.

Commonly reported Long Covid symptoms

HEART

Chest pain
Chest tightness
Heart palpitations
   or arrhythmias
Rapid heart beat
High or low blood pressure
Postural hypotension

LUNGS

Breathing difficulties
Cough

STOMACH

Abdominal pain
Nausea
Diarrhoea
Bloating
Lack of appetite
Gastro-oesophageal reflux
   disease (GERD)
New or worsening allergies
   or food sensitivities

REPRODUCTIVE ORGANS

Menstrual changes
Testicular pain
Erectile dysfunction
   or loss of libido

HEAD

Tinnitus
Sore throat
Chronic congestion
   or runny nose
Headache / migraine
Dizziness
Lightheadedness
Earache
Vision problems
Sinus pain
Dizziness
Loss of taste / smell
Excessive thirst or
   dry mouth
Depression / anxiety
Lack of confidence
Low mood
Hair loss
Cognitive disruptions
   (brain fog, lack of
   concentration, memory loss)
Increased sensitivity to
   light or sound

SKIN

Skin rashes
Hives
Itchiness

ADDITIONAL SYMPTOMS

Fatigue
Fever / chills
Night sweats
Bladder dysfunction
Pins and needles
Loss of stamina
Numbness or tingling in the extremities
Lymphedema (swelling in the limbs)

Muscle pain, weakness or tremors
Joint pain, swelling or stiffness
Sleep disturbances
Nightmares / vivid dreams
Swollen lymph nodes
Post-exertional malaise
Inability to regulate body temperature

MAIN SYMPTOMS OF LONG COVID	
Fatigue and weakness	Feeling tired and weak, even after rest or sleep. Fatigue can manifest as a persistent feeling of exhaustion, interfering with daily activities. Some individuals may also experience muscle weakness or difficulty with coordination.
Shortness of breath	Difficulty breathing or tightness in the chest, even with mild exertion, can persist after recovering from acute COVID-19. This sensation can be accompanied by other symptoms such as fatigue and cough.
Chest pain	Chest pain or discomfort may be a persistent symptom. It can vary in intensity and may be accompanied by shortness of breath or fatigue.
Muscle or joint pain	Soreness, stiffness or achiness in the muscles or joints are commonly reported. The pain can be localised or felt throughout the body, impacting physical activity and mobility.
Headaches	Persistent headaches, ranging from dull aches to throbbing pains, which can be accompanied by sensitivity to light or sound.
Loss of smell or taste	Loss of smell or taste can occur in Long Covid. It can be temporary or persistent, and may affect a person's ability to enjoy food and detect certain odours.
Cognitive difficulties	Long Covid patients may experience cognitive difficulties, often described as 'brain fog'. These can affect memory, concentration and clear thinking, causing frustration and challenges in daily tasks.
Sleep disturbances	Sleep issues are common and may include difficulty falling asleep, staying asleep or poor sleep quality. Sleep disturbances can exacerbate other symptoms such as fatigue and cognitive difficulties.
Anxiety or depression	Mental health issues, such as anxiety and depression, may persist in some individuals. Ongoing worry, fear, sadness or loss of interest in activities can be part of these experiences.

Do any of these symptoms feel familiar? For example, if you've had ME/ CFS in the past, you may experience an exacerbation of your previous symptoms such as post-exertional malaise (PEM) and extreme fatigue. You may also be experiencing some or all of the symptoms across the different body systems. While I never lost my taste or smell and didn't have any gastrointestinal disturbances (a good thing because I write gut-health recipe books!), I did have pericarditis, chest pain, peripheral neuropathy and tachycardia.

Diagnosing Long Covid

The diagnostic criteria for Long Covid include a history of COVID-19 or vaccination, symptoms persisting for 12 or more weeks, no alternative diagnosis and significant impact on daily life. Diagnosis relies on clinical evaluation and medical history, and research is ongoing into improving the diagnostic criteria and identifying specific biomarkers. Please visit superchargedfood.com/longcovid for a list of specific tests.

LONG COVID DIAGNOSIS TESTS

✦ Blood tests evaluate inflammation and immune response.

✦ Imaging tests check for lung, brain and abdominal abnormalities.

✦ Pulmonary function tests assess lung function and oxygen levels.

✦ Neurocognitive assessments test cognitive function and 'brain fog'.

✦ Cardiac evaluations examine heart function and abnormalities.

The role of autophagy in Long Covid

I like to think of autophagy as the process of our cells cleaning up their own mess, like the Marie Kondo of the cellular world. Autophagy is the ultimate decluttering, encouraging our cells to go all #KonMari and discard any unnecessary junk. But what about if they've taken the phrase 'one person's trash is another person's treasure' too literally and refuse to part ways with anything? It's like an episode of *Hoarders*, in which our cells have transformed into microscopic collectors, accumulating all sorts of cellular curiosities and hanging on to them for dear life. This peculiar phenomenon mirrors a potential mechanism implicated in Long Covid: autophagy dysfunction. Just as the hoarders in the show struggle to let go of their possessions, our cells with compromised autophagy find themselves holding on tightly to cellular components they should discard.

Several studies have found autophagy dysfunction in patients with severe COVID-19,[15] which may contribute to the disease. For example, autophagy dysfunction has been linked to misfolded proteins and damaged mitochondria building up in cells, both of which have been implicated in COVID-19. It has also been linked to a dysregulated immune response to viral infections, which may contribute to the development of Long Covid. Autophagy dysfunction may be involved in some of the hallmark symptoms of Long Covid, such as fatigue and muscle weakness, through impaired muscle function and mitochondrial dysfunction.

One 2023 study[16] investigated the role of autophagy in COVID-19 and Long Covid. It found that autophagy dysfunction may contribute to the development of Long Covid, and that therapies targeting autophagy could potentially treat this condition.

Viral loads and viral responses

Like that uninvited friend who overstays their welcome, viruses can lead to a wide range of symptoms, from mild sniffles to severe fevers. 'Viral load' refers to the amount of a virus in an infected person's body, and helps to determine a disease's infectiousness and severity.

Various factors influence an individual's viral load. Early-stage infections usually show higher viral loads that decrease as the immune response kicks in. A person's severity of infection, age, sex and underlying health conditions also affect the viral load. High viral loads can overwhelm the immune system, causing severe symptoms and complications, while lower loads mean the immune system can better control the infection.

As mentioned, the primary target for SARS-CoV-2 is ACE2, a protein on host cell surfaces. The immune response has innate and adaptive mechanisms that recognise and neutralise the virus. Some individuals may experience an autoimmune response, however, in which the immune system mistakenly attacks the body.

Older adults, and those with health issues such as asthma or autoimmune disorders, are at higher risk of severe symptoms and Long Covid. Genes also impact the disease severity, with certain gene variants increasing a person's susceptibility.

New virus variants may alter the presentation and severity of the disease, further affecting the body's response to COVID-19 and Long Covid. We need to understand these factors to manage the impact of the virus and develop targeted treatments for those affected.

Chinks in your armour and past health issues

As a clinical nutritionist, I've always been fascinated by medical mysteries. When I contracted Long Covid myself and saw the havoc it wreaked on people's lives, I knew I had to uncover its enigmas. In my quest for answers, I used myself as a human guinea pig to delve into the mysteries of Long Covid. I spoke to numerous people who were experiencing similar symptoms to those they'd had in the past, like fatigue, muscle or joint pain and cognitive difficulties.

I was eager to ascertain whether pre-existing health conditions could worsen or become more challenging to manage due to the virus's long-term effects. It was then I had a lightbulb moment. Long Covid has the power to reignite people's past health issues.

Because it's characterised by persistent symptoms that can last for weeks or months after the acute illness has resolved, they can be similar to symptoms experienced during previous illnesses. It is also opportunistic, exacerbating pre-existing conditions by taking advantage of any weaknesses or vulnerabilities in the body's immune system or other systems.

I was keen to understand what this opportunistic nature meant during my own recovery period. Imagine for a moment that you're in an episode of your favourite home-renovation show. You've just started renovating a house, fixing some longstanding problem areas. Everything is fitted in the bathroom; the paint is drying; it's almost done. Suddenly, a builder comes in with a stand-up drill – your newly perfect bathroom is now a mess. You turn to your left, and the kitchen's being bulldozed by a different builder.

Long Covid can be ruthless, and it likes to travel – its search-and-destroy function is second to none. Imagine a high-tech radar that locates your past problems, or as I like to call them, the 'chinks in your armour'. Once located, it sends in a wrecking ball to reactivate those pesky issues

When Long Covid says,
'I'm back, baby!',
all you need to do is say,
'So am I!'

you thought you'd left behind. It's like, 'Surprise! I'm back, baby!' The worst part is, you might not even notice it at first. But then, slowly but surely, those old symptoms start creeping back in.

People tell countless stories of how their past demons resurfaced with a vengeance after contracting Long Covid. For some, it's glandular fever making a comeback. For others, it's their periods going haywire. And for me? Well, chronic fatigue and mast cell activation are back on the menu – and this time, they've brought a chainsaw!

Why does this occur? First, COVID-19 infection can lead to a dysregulation of the immune system, which means existing health problems can flare up or become more severe. Second, the inflammation and damage caused by a COVID-19 infection and subsequent diagnosis of Long Covid can exacerbate existing or past health problems. The spike protein can also hide in reservoirs in the body, keeping you in the inflammatory and reactionary immune dysregulation cycle.

In some cases, Long Covid may not just lead a flare-up of an existing health problem, but rather a persistence of the initial symptoms of COVID-19 infection. For example, someone who experienced fatigue and brain fog during their COVID-19 infection may find these symptoms persisting for months – or even years – after the initial infection has resolved.

Australian National University virologist Brett Lidbury, who researches post-viral fatigue syndromes, believes Long Covid is the post-viral form of ME/CFS. He says that 30 years of research into post-viral fatigue could give scientists 'a massive head-start' in understanding Long Covid.[17]

Recent studies suggest a link between COVID-19 infection and a reactivation of the Epstein–Barr virus (EBV),[18] which causes glandular fever (also known as infectious mononucleosis).

EBV, a member of the herpesvirus family, can remain dormant in the body for years after an initial infection. Certain factors, such as a weakened immune system and inflammation from other infections like COVID-19, can cause the virus to reactivate, leading to symptoms such as fatigue, muscle aches and fever.[19]

Individuals with Long Covid often show elevated levels of EBV antibodies.[20] Some studies have found that Long Covid patients with a prior history of EBV infection had a higher risk of developing Long Covid symptoms.[21] When the notorious EBV virus hit the rewind button for me and paid another visit during Long Covid, it felt like I had enrolled in the School of Exhaustion. Fatigue, swollen glands and overall malaise became constant companions, making every step feel like a marathon and every task an uphill battle.

Mast cells and MCAS

Scientists believe contracting COVID-19 can lead to the increase of MCAS[22] or may exaggerate existing symptoms. MCAS is where mast cells (a kind of white blood cell) release histamine to fight off infection in response to a foreign substance in your body. This can lead to something called a cytokine storm, where the body produces inflammatory cytokines (these are proteins essential in cell signalling).[22] The excessive production of cytokines leads to the aggravation of cells and tissues and widespread tissue damage.

After spending weeks battling COVID-19 in the UK, I finally returned home to recover. But just when I thought I was on the mend, a not-so-new affliction struck.

My MCAS, which had been dormant for so long, flared up with a vengeance. I was still fatigued and struggling with brain fog, but now my skin felt like it was crawling with tiny insects. The constant itchiness and prickliness were unbearable. I found myself scratching at my skin until it bled. As if that wasn't bad enough, I developed hives all over my body, each one angrier and more inflamed than the last. My eyes became a constant source of irritation, weeping uncontrollably like a dripping tap.

Despite my best efforts to manage these symptoms, my body would sometimes rebel against me, throwing me into a state of misery. I was trapped in a never-ending cycle of pain and frustration.

As I recounted my symptoms, I went over the timelines. I realised I had experienced changes in my mast cell symptoms since contracting the virus. This gave me my 'light bulb moment'. There had been a definite increase in my symptoms since my bout with COVID-19. The fatigue and brain fog had been compounded by the relentless itching, hives and watering eyes. Because the virus can trigger a cascade of inflammatory responses in the body, it made my existing MCAS symptoms worse.

From revelation to relief, I was finally putting the jigsaw pieces of this complex relationship together. This was why my symptoms had been so severe, and why they seemed to be getting worse rather than better. Sometimes, even in the midst of adversity, you can have moments of clarity and insight. This was a turning point in my journey towards recovery.

As previously outlined, Long Covid is the result of an overactive immune response to SARS-CoV-2, which leads to chronic inflammation and tissue damage. Mast cells, which are located in tissues and organs like the lungs, skin and gut, play a critical role in regulating inflammation and repairing tissues.

Mast cells are activated by viral infections, releasing molecules, such as histamine, cytokines and chemokines, in response. While this response is essential to clear viral pathogens, excessive or prolonged mast cell activation can lead to tissue damage and chronic inflammation.

COVID-19 may be linked to MCAS for several reasons:

1. COVID-19 causes an immune response that can lead to the release of inflammatory molecules, including cytokines, histamine and other mediators, which activated mast cells also release). This suggests that COVID-19 infection could potentially trigger mast cell activation.

2. COVID-19 infection can cause damage to the endothelial cells that line blood vessels. This damage can increase the permeability of blood vessels, allowing mast cells to enter tissues and release their contents more easily.

3. COVID-19 infection can cause oxidative stress, which can activate mast cells and exacerbate MCAS symptoms.

4. Some individuals with MCAS experience a worsening of symptoms after contracting COVID-19.

Mast cell activation may contribute to Long Covid developing. For example, a 2021 study published in the *Journal of Allergy and Clinical Immunology*[24] found that patients with Long Covid had higher levels of tryptase, a marker of mast cell activation, than those who had recovered from COVID-19 without persistent symptoms. Another study published in *Frontiers in Medicine*[25] found that patients with Long Covid had elevated levels of cytokines and chemokines, which are released by mast cells. A further study[26] found that Long Covid patients had elevated levels of mast cell activation markers in their nasal secretions.

The exact mechanisms by which mast cells contribute to Long Covid are not yet fully understood, but there are several hypotheses. One is that mast cells may contribute to chronic inflammation and tissue damage by releasing pro-inflammatory cytokines and chemokines, such as IL-6, TNF-α and CXCL8. Another is that mast cells may damage tissues by releasing proteases, such as tryptase and chymase, that can break down extracellular matrix proteins. The virus also triggers an abnormal immune response, which leads to mast cell activation and inflammatory mediators being released.

Dr Jill Carnahan, a functional medical doctor specialising in MCAS, explains that mast cells can be triggered by viruses like SARS-CoV-2. In Long Covid, patients may experience severe mast cell activation, leading to the excessive release of histamine, cytokines and other inflammatory mediators.

COVID-19 can trigger MCAS due to an aggressive viral infection, leading to mast cell overactivity and the release of oxidating molecules. If you have a genetic predisposition to oxidative stress, you may be more susceptible to developing MCAS after COVID-19, but it's not the only factor.

Dr Carnahan also sees T-cell exhaustion, low cortisol levels and reactivation of dormant viruses in

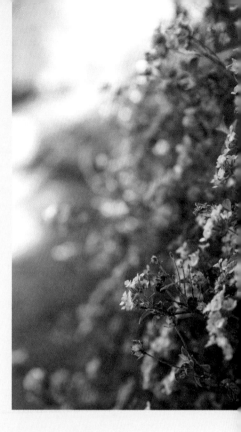

Long Covid cases, which can cause MCAS. In her clinical practice, she addresses these by treating B-cell activation, viral infections, postural tachycardia syndrome, dysautonomia, hypercoagulability and hypoxia, which leads to her patients seeing improvements.

One potential treatment approach for Long Covid uses mast cell stabilisers. These medications prevent mast cells from releasing inflammatory mediators and different types of antihistamines. They are used to treat allergies and asthma, and they may be effective in reducing mast cell activation and inflammation in COVID-19 patients with Long Covid symptoms. I have highlighted natural and food-based mast cell stabilisers in the treatment section (see pages 146–52) and low-histamine recipes (see pages 183–231) in this book.

Inflammation and Long Covid

It can be deflating when the puffiness and ache of inflammation is on your doorstep. Inflammation is a normal response of the body's immune system to infection, injury or trauma. It helps the body fight off infection and heal damaged tissues. Chronic inflammation can be harmful to the body, however; it has been linked to health problems including heart disease, diabetes and cancer.

Inflammation can also play a pivotal role in Long Covid.

COVID-19 can cause a 'cytokine storm',[27] which is an overproduction of inflammatory molecules called cytokines. This cytokine storm can damage the lungs, heart and other organs, leading to long-lasting symptoms. Some people with Long Covid have elevated levels of C-reactive protein (CRP) and interleukin-6 (IL-6), which are associated with inflammation.

Cytokines are small proteins produced by immune cells that help to regulate the immune response. An overactive immune response can lead to excessive cytokine production, or a cytokine storm. During a cytokine storm, the cytokines recruit immune cells to the site of infection, causing inflammation and tissue damage. Cytokines can also activate other cells, such as endothelial cells, which line blood vessels. This can lead to increased permeability of the blood vessels, allowing fluid and immune cells to leak into the surrounding tissues, contributing to inflammation and tissue damage.

The body has a complex immune response to a virus, which is essential for controlling and eliminating the infection but can also lead to complications. For example, in COVID-19, the immune response can cause inflammation of and damage to the lungs, leading to respiratory failure and other complications. Some individuals have a robust immune response, which is effective at clearing the virus and preventing severe disease. Others may have a weaker immune response, however, which lets the virus replicate and cause more severe symptoms. A subset of individuals may experience an overactive immune response (the cytokine storm), which is one of the key factors contributing to Long Covid.

In Long Covid, the immune system may keep producing high levels of cytokines after the initial infection has resolved. The resulting

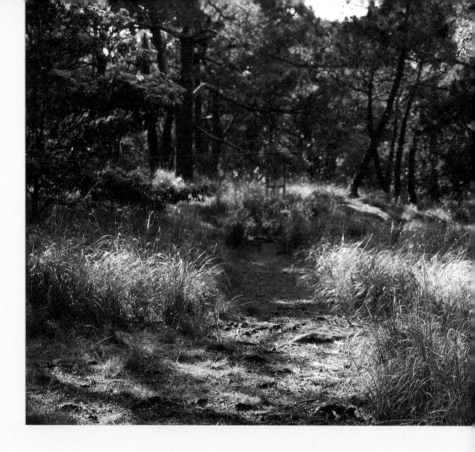

inflammation can affect multiple organ systems, including the lungs, heart, brain and gut. It can also lead to symptoms such as fatigue, brain fog, shortness of breath, chest pain, joint pain and gastrointestinal issues, which are commonly experienced by Long Covid patients.

Other factors may also contribute to inflammation in Long Covid. Long Covid patients often have imbalances in their gut microbiome, which can lead to increased inflammation in the gut and other parts of the body. Chronic stress and poor sleep can contribute to inflammation by activating the sympathetic nervous system and increasing levels of stress hormones like cortisol.

Inflammation is a complex process that plays a significant role in the symptoms of Long Covid. Understanding and targeting the mechanisms of inflammation are key to improving your health. We will cover these in Part 3: Your Long Covid support plan.

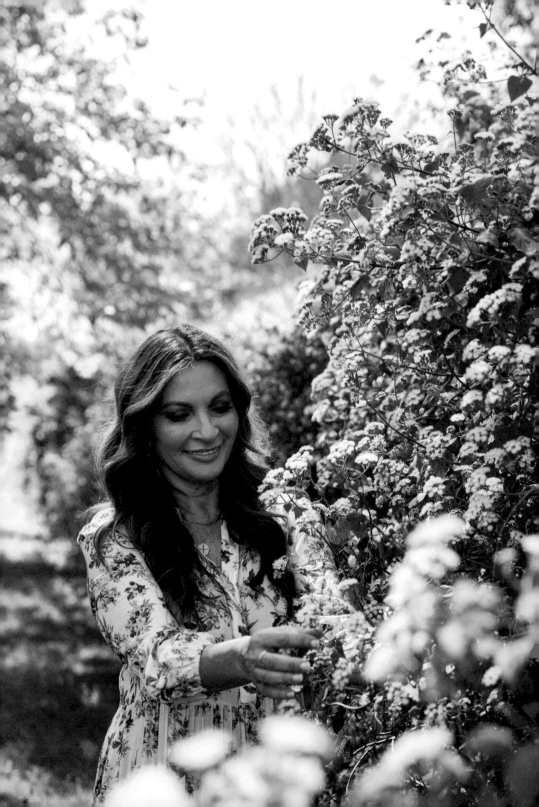

COVID-19 isn't just a respiratory problem. Beyond the breath, it touches the heart and mind, and tests our resilience.

Long Covid and your body's systems

After consulting with doctors and researchers, it became clear that each specialist had their own perspective on the main cause of Long Covid based on their area of expertise. One point of consensus among them was that underlying infections or conditions may be significant contributors to developing Long Covid.

When the COVID-19 pandemic emerged, it was initially viewed as a respiratory illness that primarily affected the lungs. This led to recommendations focused on reducing the spread of the virus through measures such as mask-wearing and social distancing, with little emphasis on other aspects of the disease. We now understand that COVID-19 is much more complex than first thought and has a range of effects beyond the respiratory system.

Although respiratory symptoms such as shortness of breath, coughing and chest pain are commonly associated with Long Covid, it can affect multiple organ systems and cause other symptoms such as fatigue, brain fog, headaches, muscle or joint pain, heart palpitations, gastrointestinal problems, and more.

While some individuals may only experience mild respiratory symptoms such as coughing and shortness of breath, others may develop severe respiratory symptoms like pneumonia. Many individuals with COVID-19 may experience non-respiratory symptoms such as fever, fatigue, headaches and loss of smell or taste. The severity of the person's initial COVID-19 infection and their immune response to the virus may impact the development and persistence of symptoms.

While the respiratory system is often the primary site of infection, COVID-19 can affect multiple body systems. This has significant implications for managing and treating the disease, as well as for understanding its long-term effects.

How Long Covid affects your body's systems

SYSTEM	SYMPTOMS
Respiratory system	Shortness of breath, coughing and chest pain
Cardiovascular system	Heart palpitations and chest pain
Nervous system	Brain fog, difficulty concentrating, memory problems and headaches
Immune system	Ongoing inflammation and autoimmune issues
Musculoskeletal system	Muscle and joint pain
Gastrointestinal system	Diarrhoea and nausea
Chemosensory system	Loss of taste and smell
Other systems	Long Covid can also affect the endocrine, renal, dermatological, ocular and auditory systems

Cardiovascular system

While most people bid farewell to their initial illness and recover, some of us are roped into an extended remix of cardiovascular symptoms after our initial bout of COVID-19. I developed pericarditis and ongoing crushing chest pain and fluttering palpitations, which took months to settle down. Finally, after what felt like an eternity of chest discomfort and rhythmic acrobatics, the symptoms took a well-deserved intermission.

Chest pain or discomfort is one of the most common, and persisting, cardiovascular symptoms of Long Covid. This may be due to ongoing inflammation in the lungs, which can lead to reduced oxygen levels and increased strain on the heart.

COVID-19 can also damage the heart muscle, resulting in a condition known as myocarditis. Myocarditis is an inflammation of the heart muscle that can weaken the heart's ability to pump blood effectively. It causes chest pain, shortness of breath and palpitations.

Another cardiovascular complication associated with COVID-19 is blood clots. COVID-19 can make the blood more prone to clotting. This can lead to deep vein thrombosis (DVT), a condition in which blood clots form in the veins of the legs or arms, and pulmonary embolism (PE), a potentially life-threatening condition in which a blood clot travels to the lungs. People with Long Covid may be at increased risk of developing blood clots due to ongoing inflammation and immune dysfunction.

COVID-19 can damage the blood vessels and endothelium, the layer of cells lining the inside of blood vessels. This can lead to endothelial dysfunction, a condition in which the blood vessels are less able to dilate and contract. Endothelial dysfunction can contribute to hypertension, atherosclerosis and other cardiovascular diseases.

As well as these cardiovascular complications, Long Covid can also cause other symptoms that may directly or indirectly affect the cardiovascular system. For example, many people with Long Covid report feeling fatigued and weak, which can make it difficult to exercise and maintain a healthy lifestyle. This can contribute to developing cardiovascular risk factors such as obesity, hypertension and diabetes. The stress and anxiety associated with Long Covid also have ripple effects on the cardiovascular system.

Because people with Long Covid may experience persistent chest pain, blood clots and endothelial dysfunction, these complications can contribute to the development of more serious cardiovascular diseases such as heart failure and stroke. Healthcare providers should be aware of the potential complications and monitor patients for any signs of cardiovascular symptoms. Lifestyle modifications such as exercise, healthy diet, stress reduction and appropriate medical management may help to mitigate the cardiovascular risks associated with Long Covid.

Understanding the cardiovascular implications

Thao Huynh, an epidemiologist and cardiologist at McGill University Health Centre in Montreal, Canada, says that scans on more than 100 Long Covid patients showed 30 per cent had signs of active inflammation around their heart and another 40 per cent had scar tissue; almost all also had elevated blood markers for inflammation.[28]

A study published in *JAMA Cardiology*[29] found that COVID-19 survivors had a higher risk of developing heart failure, ischaemic heart disease and other cardiovascular complications compared to people who did not contract the virus. The exact mechanism by which COVID-19 and Long Covid affect the cardiovascular system is still unclear. The virus may infect the heart muscle or blood vessels directly, leading to inflammation, scarring and other complications. Or perhaps the virus triggers an abnormal immune response, leading to inflammation and damage to the cardiovascular system.

One way to reduce the cardiovascular risk associated with Long Covid is to identify and treat risk factors such as hypertension, high cholesterol and diabetes, which will reduce the risk of heart disease and other cardiovascular complications.[30]

Blood clotting

Picture this: within the intricate highways of our circulatory system, a diligent traffic cop is ensuring smooth blood flow. Armed with their trusty whistles, they direct the red blood cells like a maestro. They wave the oxygen-rich vehicles through the arterial lanes, while ensuring waste-filled cells exit through the venous off-ramps. It's like a bustling metropolis where traffic flows harmoniously, ensuring every organ and tissue is nourished and happy. But sometimes they encounter a hiccup in their duties. Roadblocks in the form of blood clots can unexpectedly appear, causing a gridlock that

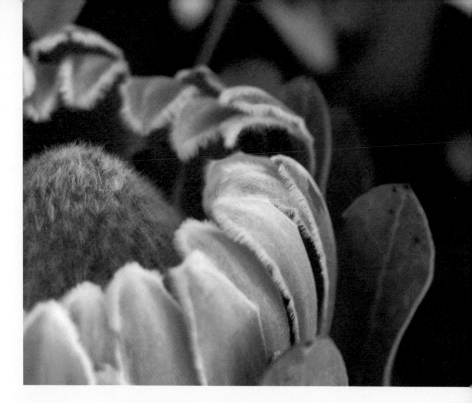

slows down the entire system. And in the case of Long Covid, those blood clots come in the form of a Mini Minor, or a microclot!

Blood clotting is an essential bodily process that stops excessive bleeding. After you get a cut, the body normally dissolves blood clots, but in certain conditions, including both acute and Long Covid, smaller clots, called microclots, don't follow regular protocol. Rather than dissolving, microclots block blood vessels and stop oxygen flowing throughout the body, causing symptoms like shortness of breath, fatigue, brain fog and even long-term organ damage.[31] Microclots may be responsible for many Long Covid symptoms.

Microclotting can occur in the lungs, heart, brain, kidneys and liver. In the lungs, it can lead to reduced oxygen uptake, which can cause shortness of breath and other respiratory symptoms.

In addition to medical treatment, you can reduce your risk of microclotting with natural anti-inflammatories and lifestyle modifications, such as exercise, healthy diet and stress reduction. You'll also improve your overall health and well-being.

Clotting and inflammatory molecules

I spoke with Dr Resia Pretorius, the head of department and a distinguished research professor in the Physiological Sciences Department, Faculty of Science, Stellenbosch University, South Africa, about coagulation, microclotting and changes in inflammatory profiles, including molecules that come via gut dysbiosis.

I asked Dr Pretorious how microclots develop and their link to acute and Long Covid patients. 'Acute Covid patients are exposed to spike protein which is the main inflammagen from the virus. During that process the spike protein comes into circulation and binds directly to the ACE2 receptors, it can also bind to platelets,' she said. 'Clots form, the protein structure changes and microclots, together with the platelet hyperactivation, interact with the endothelial layers. The microclots per se are not the causative agent of Long Covid, it is the result of the spike protein from the acute phase. In some individuals the spike protein persists for a longer period and leads to damage to the endothelial layers.

'In some patients that have genetic clotting disorders, this will take longer for the clots to break down.'

Nervous system

Long Covid has a mischievous penchant for affecting the nervous system, leading to symptoms like fatigue, brain fog, cognitive issues, headaches, sleep disturbances and pain. The nervous system can be impacted through changes in brain structure, inflammation and decreased connectivity. Dysfunction of the autonomic nervous system may also affect heart rate and blood pressure regulation.

Neurological symptoms in Long Covid could be linked to a phenomenon called 'antigenic imprinting'. This is where the immune system produces antibodies to past viral infections instead of the current threat (SARS-CoV-2). Antigenic imprinting may explain the persistent neurological symptoms experienced by individuals with Long Covid, because antibodies produced in response to previous coronaviruses may play a role.

Central nervous system

Long Covid can affect the nervous system by causing central nervous system (CNS) dysregulation. Including the brain and spinal cord, the CNS is responsible for controlling many bodily functions. COVID-19 can cause inflammation in the CNS, which can damage the neurons and disrupt normal brain function.

Symptoms of CNS dysregulation can include headaches, dizziness and cognitive impairment. Some individuals with Long Covid may also experience more severe symptoms such as seizures, encephalitis or stroke. Long Covid patients may have alterations in their brain structure and function, including reduced grey matter volume and abnormal brain activity. [32]

There are several possible mechanisms for how this happens. One is that the virus directly invades the CNS and damages the neurons and supporting cells. Another is that the body's immune response to the virus triggers an inflammatory response in the CNS, leading to damage and dysfunction.

As Dr Robert Groysman from reliefbeginshere.com explained, 'One of the many functions of the parasympathetic nervous system and the vagus nerve is to modulate the immune system and inflammation. Chronic inflammation comes directly from an activation of the immune system. During the actual infection, there is an exaggerated immune response, and it can trigger inflammation. The immune cells then release cytokines, which are mediators, to activate the immune system even more. This happens in the nervous system as well.'

COVID-19 can persist in the CNS for some time after the initial infection. One study published in *Nature* in November 2020[33] reported that SARS-CoV-2 RNA was detectable in the brain tissue of patients who died from COVID-19, suggesting that the virus can stay in the CNS.

Peripheral nervous system

The peripheral nervous system (PNS) is responsible for transmitting sensory and motor signals between the CNS and the rest of the body. COVID-19 can damage the PNS, leading to peripheral neuropathy. This is a condition that causes numbness, tingling or weakness in the extremities, such as the hands and feet. It can also cause debilitating pain or discomfort.

✳ MY EXPERIENCE WITH PERIPHERAL NEUROPATHY ✳

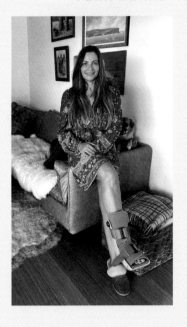

During Long Covid, I had intense peripheral neuropathy. One day, I'd taken a pew at a local café to drink chai when I experienced pins and needles in my foot. Thinking it was just a regular case of pins and needles, I gave my leg a good shake, ready to carry on with my day. But Long Covid had other plans in store. As I took my first steps, my right leg felt like a plate of jiggly jelly, betraying my sense of balance. When I put it down on the concrete floor, I could not feel my foot or leg anymore. My knee gave way (it had been injured in a car accident earlier in the year) and my body crumpled to the floor, rolling my ankle in the process. Ouch!

As I lay there, contemplating my next move, I saw that my foot had undergone a transformation worthy of a deep sea creature from folklore, swelling up like a puffer fish. I caught a glimpse of myself in a nearby shop window. I resembled none other than Bigfoot, sasquatching my way to the nearest doctor's surgery for tests and answers.

Over the coming days, my foot and toes turned black. I was in excruciating pain. The test came back revealing it was broken in two places: the calcaneus or heel bone, the largest bone in the foot, and the talus bone, at the top of the foot. I also had two ligament tears. Spending Easter holidays in a moon boot was not my idea of fun. Instead of hunting for colourful eggs, I hobbled through the season, a bittersweet reminder that life has a peculiar way of serving up unexpected challenges.

People with Long Covid may have a higher risk of developing peripheral neuropathy than those who have not experienced acute COVID-19.[34] Patients with COVID-19 have also reported nerve pain and skeletal muscle injury, Guillain-Barré syndrome, cranial polyneuritis, neuromuscular junction disorders, neuro-ophthalmological disorders, neurosensory hearing loss and dysautonomia.[35]

Long Covid may be associated with an increased risk of developing small fibre neuropathy,[36] a type of peripheral neuropathy that affects the small nerve fibres responsible for transmitting sensory and autonomic signals from the skin and organs to the brain. It can cause symptoms such as pain, burning, tingling, and numbness in the hands, feet and other areas of the body. Vitamin B12 and other nutrients are essential for nerve health; include these in a balanced diet to help with symptoms. Acupuncture, warm baths and stress-management techniques like meditation and yoga may also alleviate symptoms.

Autonomic nervous system

The autonomic nervous system (ANS) is a behind-the-scenes hero, a backstage director diligently managing our body's involuntary functions. Picture this: the ANS takes charge of our heart rate, keeping it in rhythm like a conductor leading an orchestra. The ANS also directs our blood pressure, ensuring a tightrope-walker's delicate balance, navigating the highs and lows. It is an expert in controlling each inhale and exhale of our breath. The ANS works tirelessly to keep our bodily functions humming along smoothly, even when we're blissfully unaware of its intricate choreography.

COVID-19 can lead to dysregulation of the ANS, known as autonomic dysfunction. Symptoms of autonomic dysfunction include changes in heart rate or blood pressure, difficulty regulating body temperature and gastrointestinal symptoms. Long Covid patients may experience autonomic dysfunction for weeks or months after their initial infection. One study found that nearly 80 per cent of Long Covid patients reported symptoms such as rapid heart rate or palpitations, while 42 per cent reported gastrointestinal symptoms.[37] Patients with Long Covid often experience symptoms related to dysautonomia (a condition where the ANS doesn't function properly), including palpitations, dizziness, fainting, shortness of breath and gastrointestinal problems.[38]

Neuroinflammation

As well as the direct effects of COVID-19 on the nervous system, the body's immune response to the virus can cause neuroinflammation. In neuroinflammation, the immune system responds to an injury or infection in the CNS by sending immune cells and inflammatory molecules to the affected area.

COVID-19 can cause neuroinflammation in the brain and other parts of the nervous system,[39] leading to neurological symptoms such as cognitive impairment, fatigue and mood changes. Long Covid patients may have elevated levels of inflammatory markers in the blood and cerebrospinal fluid, indicating that their immune response to the virus may be contributing to neuroinflammation.

Psychiatric symptoms

Long Covid has extended into the realms of our mental well-being, leading to psychiatric symptoms including anxiety, depression and post-traumatic stress disorder (PTSD). As if the physical challenges weren't enough, Long Covid throws a psychological curveball into the mix as it ventures into the intricate landscapes of our minds.

During my journey with Long Covid, I found myself becoming a seeker of light in the darkest corners. Most days, I carried a flickering candle of hope, determined to illuminate even the tiniest glimmers of positivity. When fatigue threatened to engulf me in suffocating darkness, I mustered every ounce of strength to defy its grasp. When brain fog clouded my thoughts, I kept searching for moments of clarity. When waves of uncertainty crashed upon my shores, I clung to the belief that brighter days were just beyond the horizon. Long Covid tested my endurance, but it couldn't extinguish my flame of determination. I had beaten MCAS and ME/CFS in the past, so I knew I could beat this. With unwavering resolve, I ventured into the depths, unafraid of the shadows. I knew that amidst the gloom, a spark of light would guide me forward.

And I did find glimpses of joy, pockets of gratitude. I knew that I wasn't alone: Long Covid sufferers are at increased risk of developing psychiatric symptoms. The stress of being ill with COVID-19, the fear of potential complications or death and the social isolation and economic stressors associated with the pandemic can all contribute to developing psychiatric symptoms.

We've already seen how the virus can affect the nervous system, leading to dysregulation and psychiatric symptoms. COVID-19 can cause inflammation in the CNS, which can damage neurons and disrupt normal brain function, contributing to psychiatric symptoms developing.

For many people, coping with anxiety related to Long Covid is an ongoing process, which I will cover in more detail in Part 2: Hold on. Help is on its way (see pages 63–140). Being committed to prioritising mental health and well-being is an important step in your recovery.

Immune system

As we've discussed, the immune system is the body's defence mechanism against foreign invaders such as viruses and bacteria. It is composed of specialised cells such as T cells, B cells and natural killer cells, which work together to identify and destroy pathogens.

During a viral infection, the immune system mobilises an army of immune cells to detect and destroy the invading virus. This response controls the infection and prevents the virus from spreading throughout the body. In some cases, however, the immune response can become overly aggressive, leading to excessive inflammation and tissue damage called the 'cytokine storm'.

In the beginning of the pandemic, much attention was focused on harmful inflammation and cytokine storms in severe COVID-19 patients. Researchers soon discovered antibodies were targeting the patient's own body rather than attacking SARS-CoV-2, the virus responsible for COVID-19. Individuals with severe COVID-19 were exhibiting similar characteristics to those with chronic autoimmune disorders, in which the immune system attacks the body's own tissues.

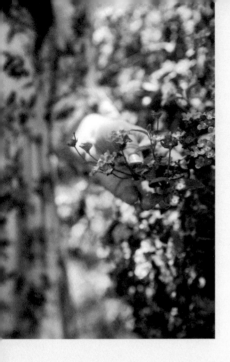

Matthew Woodruff, Instructor of Human Immunology at Emory University in Atlanta, USA, is part of a team that has been investigating the connection between COVID-19 and autoimmunity. In their recent publication in *Nature*, the researchers uncovered that, in severe COVID-19 cases, many of the antibodies that neutralise the virus also attack the patient's own organs and tissues. These self-targeting antibodies can persist for months or even years in Long Covid patients, highlighting the connection between antiviral immunity and chronic autoimmune diseases.

By understanding the immune system's role in Long Covid, we can gain insights into potential treatment strategies. Therapies that modulate the immune system's response, for instance, may be effective in treating Long Covid. These aim to reduce inflammation and restore balance to the immune system, potentially improving symptoms and reducing the risk of long-term complications.

Other treatments include oxygen therapy, physiotherapy and cognitive-behavioural therapy. These aim to address the symptoms and complications associated with Long Covid, including fatigue, shortness of breath, muscle weakness and cognitive difficulties.

Immune dysfunction may play a role in the persistent hypoxemia some individuals with Long Covid have. Hypoxemia is a condition characterised by low oxygen levels in the blood, which can cause shortness of breath, fatigue and other symptoms. Oxygen therapy may help patients who experience persistent hypoxemia. This therapy involves delivering oxygen to the patient either through a nasal cannula or face mask. By helping to increase oxygen levels in the blood, it can improve symptoms and promote healing.

The book includes a section on protocols with holistic steps you can take to support your immune system and improve overall health (see pages 159–60). Some steps include maintaining a healthy, nutrient-rich diet, staying physically active within your limits, managing stress through techniques such as meditation or deep breathing exercises, getting enough sleep and avoiding harmful habits such as smoking and drinking too much alcohol.

Musculoskeletal system

Comprising of bones, muscles, ligaments, tendons and other connective tissues, the musculoskeletal system literally supports the body, letting us move and maintain our posture. The bones provide structure, protect organs and store minerals, while the muscles allow for voluntary and involuntary movement. Ligaments and tendons stabilise joints and connect muscles to bones. We need a healthy musculoskeletal system to perform daily activities and for our overall well-being.

Long Covid can impact the musculoskeletal system in various ways. Some patients report persistent symptoms, including muscle weakness, joint pain and fatigue. Muscle weakness can result from inactivity during the illness's acute phase as well as inflammation of muscles or nerves, or autoimmune responses affecting the muscles. This weakness can hamper daily activities like walking and lifting.

Joint pain and inflammation, another common complaint, is triggered by the immune system's response to the virus. Long Covid may lead to autoimmune disorders like rheumatoid arthritis, contributing to joint discomfort.

Fatigue, a prevalent symptom, can stem from the virus itself or the body's immune response. Long Covid fatigue can feel like overwhelming and unending exhaustion, similar to the Greek myth of Sisyphus endlessly pushing a boulder uphill. Individuals battle constant fatigue to manage symptoms and maintain normalcy in their lives.

Along with muscle and joint pain and fatigue, Long Covid patients might experience postural orthostatic tachycardia syndrome (POTS), which is characterised by abnormal increases in heart rate upon posture changes. POTS can cause dizziness, fainting and fatigue, and further impact the musculoskeletal system by weakening muscles and causing pain.

Managing Long Covid's impact on the musculoskeletal system requires rest, pacing, rehabilitation, physiotherapy and exercise when feasible. These measures can enhance your muscle strength, joint flexibility and endurance over time. While the road to recovery might be arduous, resilience and persistence will help you strive for a better quality of life.

Gastrointestinal system

Post-Covid belly can really get you down. Some people experience lingering digestive issues after contracting COVID-19. I've seen a wealth of post-Covid gut issues in my nutritional clinic – from bloating, reflux and flatulence to constipation, diarrhoea, dysbiosis and leaky gut syndrome.

The gut is the body's epicentre of health. It's central to many bodily systems, including the immune system, so it isn't surprising that the aftermath of COVID-19 can come in the form of digestive issues and complications.

Common gut symptoms associated with the virus include vomiting, diarrhoea, constipation, a lack of appetite, abdominal pain, flatulence, distorted taste and nausea. If you're experiencing any of these during or after catching COVID-19, you're not alone. Up to one-third of people with COVID-19 have experienced gastrointestinal symptoms.

So why and how does COVID-19 impact the gut?

I spoke with Dr Vincent Pedre, a board-certified internist and functional medicine practitioner from New York, USA, who believes we can find answers by looking at the gut microbiome of centenarians. He confirmed, 'the gut microbiome in centenarians has certain resilience factors such as protection against infection or the ability to reduce inflammation when it occurs. Those that age rapidly will tend to have an ageing microbiome that over time is going to favour more inflammation in the body. So if we transfer it into why certain people develop Long Covid versus why others don't, we know that certain people just don't resolve inflammation.'

Inflammation is one of the key drivers of Long Covid. Some people's microbiomes can protect them against infection or the ability to reduce inflammation, but other microbiomes don't have this ability.

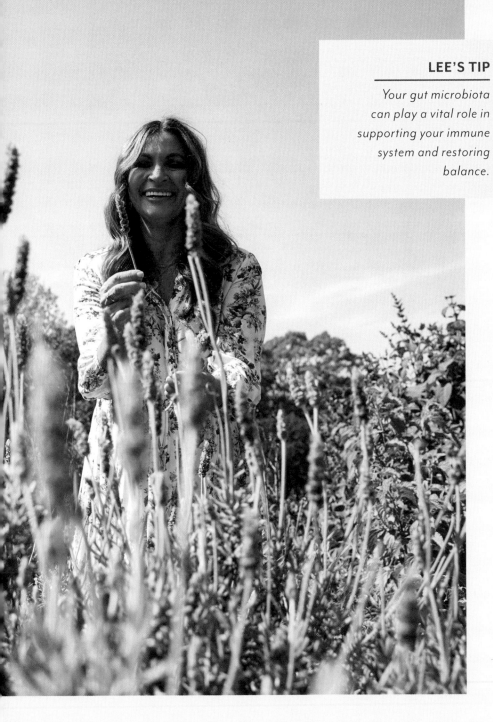

LEE'S TIP

Your gut microbiota can play a vital role in supporting your immune system and restoring balance.

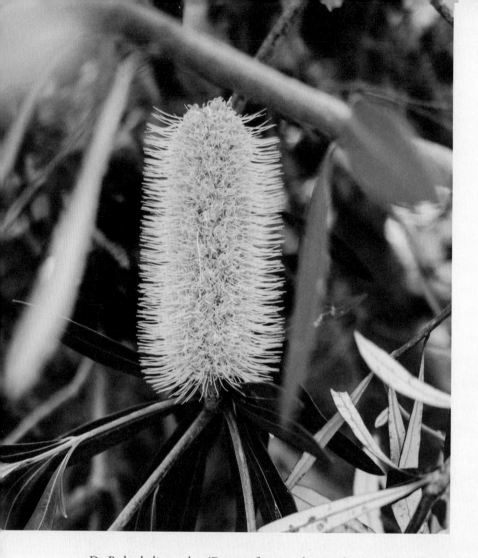

Dr Pedre believes that 'Every infectious disease that becomes chronic for people has at the root, a dysregulation of the immune system. The immune system becomes chronically activated but at the same time, the immune system is failing to recognise that the infection is gone and that it needs to turn off now, or it's not knowing how to resolve the remaining parts of infection.'

Of the spike protein, which I've highlighted in previous chapters, and its implications for the gut, Dr Pedre says, 'What we know is that there is persistence of the spike protein, and research is ongoing to ascertain if there is a viral reservoir that is the force of the spike protein. The spike protein is known to circulate in the blood in vesicles, which are small structures that can protect it from the immune system's detection and attack.'

The spike protein can be detected in stool samples of individuals infected with COVID-19,[40] and it can persist in faecal matter for up to seven months after infection. Testing for the spike protein in stool samples may provide a useful diagnostic tool for COVID-19, particularly in cases where other testing methods have yielded inconclusive or negative results.

The gut is critical to our immune system; its large and diverse population of bacteria affects the body's immune responses. Microbiome imbalances and inflammation may be implicated in Long Covid.[41]

The composition of the gut microbiota can indicate disease severity and immune responses dysfunction. Individuals with COVID-19 have fewer gut bacteria with immune-modulating properties, such as *Faecalibacterium prausnitzii*, *Eubacterium rectale* and species of *Bifidobacteria*.[42] These bacteria are responsible for producing short-chain fatty acids, which our bodies need to help reduce inflammatory cytokines and disease severity. Even after the virus has been cleared, COVID-19 patients can still have a disrupted gut microbiota, which could potentially contribute to long-lasting symptoms.

> **GUT MICROBIOME IMBALANCES AND INFLAMMATION.** This could be contributing to the persistent symptoms some individuals with Long Covid experience. By supporting a healthy gut microbiome, you could improve your immune function and potentially reduce the severity and duration of COVID-19 symptoms. A recent study links Long Covid to gut inflammation and serotonin deficiency,[43] where patients can exhibit reduced circulating levels of the neurotransmitter serotonin. Researchers discovered that some Long Covid patients had SARS-CoV-2 virus lingering in their stool samples for months after initial infection. They had a viral reservoir in the gut that triggered the immune system to release interferons. These interferons cause inflammation that hampers the gut absorption of tryptophan, a critical precursor for neurotransmitters like serotonin. Serotonin,

which is primarily produced in the gut, regulates various bodily functions, including memory, sleep, digestion and wound healing. When tryptophan absorption is disrupted due to viral inflammation in Long Covid patients, serotonin levels are depleted, affecting vagus nerve signalling and contributing to symptoms such as memory loss.

ABDOMINAL PAIN. Often reported by Long Covid patients, this can be caused by inflammation in the digestive system. This results from the immune system's response to the virus.

DIARRHOEA. This can be caused by inflammation in the intestines, which can disrupt the normal functioning of the digestive system. In some cases, bacterial overgrowth in the intestines may cause diarrhoea, especially if the gut microbiome has changed following a viral infection or there is a pre-existing imbalance.

REDUCED APPETITE. Some Long Covid patients report a significant reduction in their appetite. This can be caused by the virus itself, as well as by the immune system's response to it. Persistent loss of appetite can lead to weight loss and malnutrition.

GASTROESOPHAGEAL REFLUX DISEASE. Patients may experience gastro-oesophageal reflux disease (GERD), a condition in which stomach acid flows back into the oesophagus, causing heartburn and other symptoms. The virus's effect on the digestive system can exacerbate GERD and cause significant discomfort and disruption to daily life.

All this had me wondering, why would I suffer so heavily from peripheral neuropathy and not have any gut issues during Long Covid? When looking at the mechanisms of the disease, however, even though they are the same, in chronic conditions such as Long Covid the way it expresses itself in different people *is* different.

Nutritionally, focusing on a low-histamine gut-friendly diet filled with omega-3 fatty acids, fruits, vegetables, soups and smoothies can help. Eating foods high in polyphenols (plant-based compounds) will help to improve the mucus layer of the gut and regulate the immune system. A gut-friendly shopping list should include anti-inflammatory turmeric, gut-healing gelatine, omega-3-rich fish, protein, gut-loving supplements and a synbiotic powder to help repair, restore and rebalance your gut health from within (for more on protocols, see pages 159–60).

✳ CROSS-REACTIVITY – WHEN THE BODY REACTS TO ITSELF ✳

Some people may experience persistent symptoms because their immune system continues to attack the body even after the virus has been cleared.

Remember the spike protein? It's the part of the virus that lets it enter human cells and infect them. When the immune system detects the virus, it creates antibodies that target the spike protein to neutralise the virus. However, these antibodies may also cross-react with other tissues in the body, leading to an autoimmune response and damaging those tissues. There is evidence of cross-reactivity between the spike protein and neurological tissue, which could explain why some individuals with Long Covid experience neuropathy or other neurological symptoms – hence my peripheral neuropathy!

One potential treatment for this autoimmune response is intravenous immunoglobulin (IVIG) therapy. This treatment involves infusing antibodies from donated blood plasma into a patient's bloodstream. The donor antibodies will help to regulate the patient's immune response and reduce the autoimmune attack on their own tissues.

IVIG has been used to treat several autoimmune and inflammatory diseases, and could potentially treat Long Covid. The treatment has immune-modulating effects and may help to restore a healthy balance of gut bacteria in patients with Long Covid whose microbiota are out of balance. IVIG may also help to reduce gut inflammation, a contributor to the persistent symptoms some individuals with Long Covid experience.

Chemosensory system

Losing your sense of taste and smell can be a bitter pill to swallow. Or maybe it's sweet? It's difficult for long-haulers to tell sometimes. The percentage of people who experience loss of taste and/or smell with Long Covid can vary, but it's generally a whopping 50–70 per cent. Losing your sense of taste and smell can be perplexing and disheartening. You're left in a world of culinary confusion where flavours are indistinguishable and scents non-existent.

The chemosensory system, which is responsible for taste and smell, includes specialised cells on the tongue and in the nasal cavity. The taste buds detect sweet, sour, salty, bitter and umami flavours, while the olfactory receptors identify thousands of different smells. When Long Covid strikes these systems go on holiday, leaving the patient with a dry mouth and ineffective nose.

Anosmia, or loss of taste and smell, affects up to 80 per cent of people infected with COVID-19. While most people recover these senses within weeks, Long Covid patients may endure prolonged anosmia for several months or even longer. The precise mechanism behind this phenomenon remains elusive, but theories point to an immune response causing inflammation or direct viral damage to the olfactory tissue.

Some individuals may experience changes in their perception of taste and smell, with distorted or heightened senses. Fortunately, the body's magical stem cells in the nasal cavity can regenerate into new olfactory receptors over time, leading to potential recovery.

When treating a lost sense of smell, doctors don't have many options. It's not like they can just ask a patient to wear a peg on their nose and call it a day. Instead, they may suggest something called olfactory retraining. This involves huffing four different scents twice a day for several months – usually rose, eucalyptus, lemon and clove. It's like aromatherapy, but instead of feeling relaxed, you're just hoping your sense of smell comes back.

✳ TAMING LONG COVID ✳

Long Covid is like a circus ringmaster, juggling multiple systems in your body at once! But don't worry, I've got some tricks up my sleeve to tame those wild symptoms of yours.

In Part 2 of this book, I'll be sharing my secrets for easing common issues caused by Long Covid, healing them and decreasing their lifespan. In Parts 3 and 4, I'll reveal how to shorten the duration of Long Covid and get to the root of the problem. I'll also share 30 mouth-watering low-histamine recipes with you, so you can finally say goodbye to those pesky symptoms and get back to living your best life!

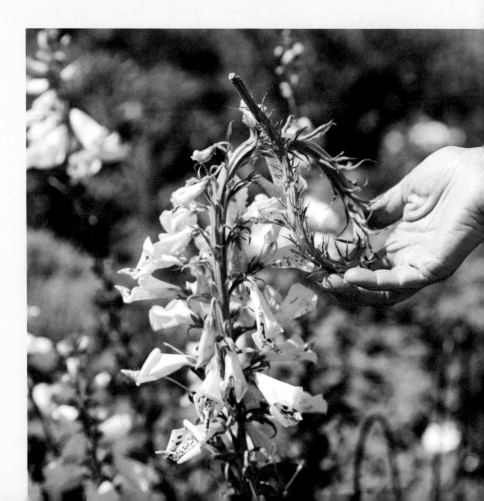

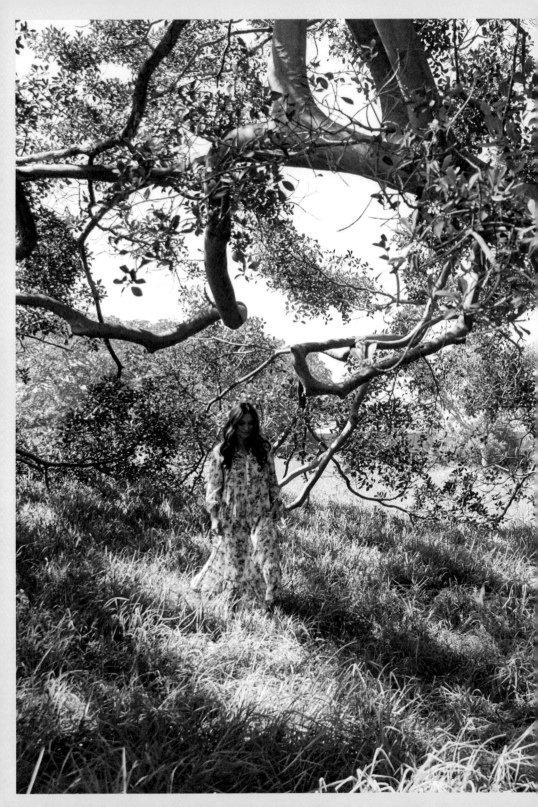

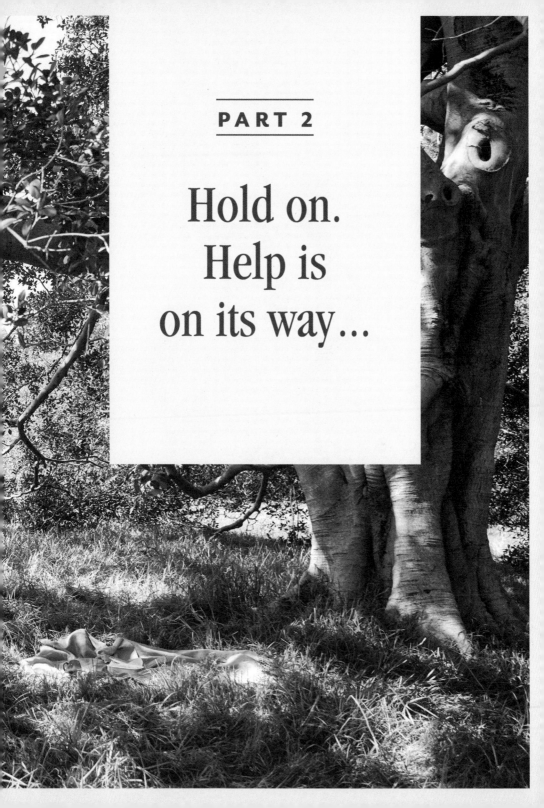

PART 2

Hold on. Help is on its way...

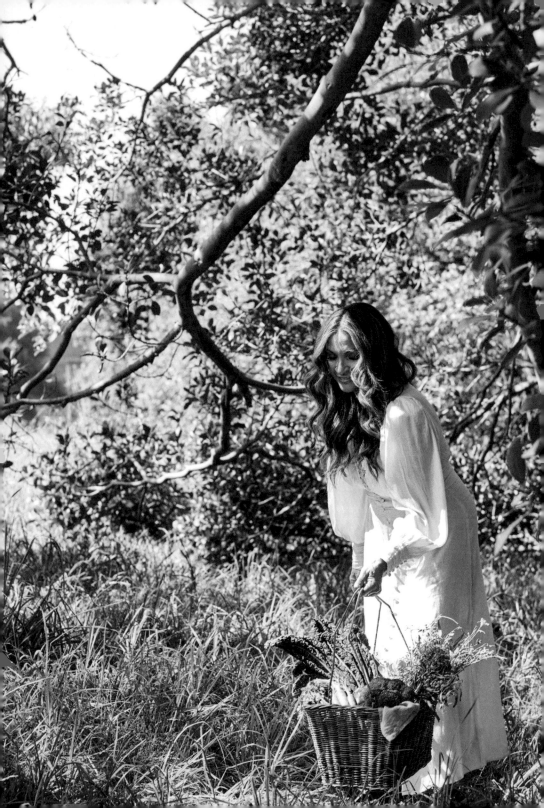

The burden of Long Covid goes beyond the physical. Share your vulnerability because it holds the key to connection and understanding.

Isolation and mental health in Long Covid

Not only can Long Covid cause physical symptoms but it can also lead to social isolation, which can have a significant impact on your mental health. Many long-haulers report feeling disconnected from their support systems and are unable to take part in social activities due to ongoing symptoms such as fatigue and brain fog.

In the darkest days of my illness, I was confined to my bed, trapped in a barely functioning body. The simplest movements left me gasping for air, and leaving the house was a long-lost dream. Day after day, I lay there in one position like a soldier who had returned from battle. In my head I felt the weight of hopelessness crushing down on me. At certain points every breath was a struggle. Every moment within those breaths was a reminder of my own fragility.

The days passed like an eternity as I lay there, my arm locked rigidly by my side and chest pressed into the bed. Every time I drew breath was like a knife piercing through my chest, sending waves of pain through my body. The agony was unbearable. Moving was out of the question. I was reminded of my past run-in with chronic fatigue, when I was trapped in my body, unable to escape the torment. It was my lowest point, and the fear of never recovering crept in. I was in a new reality – alone, helpless, consumed by the endless cycle of illness and wondering if I would ever recover.

The burden of Long Covid goes beyond the physical symptoms. It can be a lonely and isolating place. People who are battling with the aftermath of COVID-19 may face discrimination and stigma because of a lack of understanding about the prolonged effects of the virus. This judgment can make them feel ashamed and embarrassed; they may retreat from sharing their experiences or seeking support. It's not just a virus; it's a struggle against social ostracism and emotional pain.

Long Covid can create a host of physical limitations that make it nearly impossible to engage in social activities or even leave the house. The result? A deep solitude and lonesomeness that can feel all-consuming. Being unable to do the things you once enjoyed can be crushing, leaving you to feel like a shell of your former self.

The uncertainty of it all only compounds the problem. The unpredictable symptoms and lack of knowledge about Long Covid can leave you feeling like no one understands what you're going through. It's enough to make you want to hide away from the world and give up hope.

✳ CASE STUDY: LIZ ✳

Lizzie Williamson, a 45-year-old fitness educator and keynote speaker, faced shame due to Long Covid. Initially unaware of her condition, she struggled with the constant exhaustion, longing for sleep and lacking motivation. Despite fulfilling her speaking engagements with energy, she inevitably crashed afterwards. The mental toll became evident; she experienced depression and a sense of darkness.

Confiding in a friend about her struggles, however, lifted the burden of shame. By sharing her experience, she realised she was not alone. Lizzie could show herself some kindness and accept her need for rest. Sharing and releasing the shame improved her mental well-being, and her symptoms gradually improved, although occasional fatigue still persists.

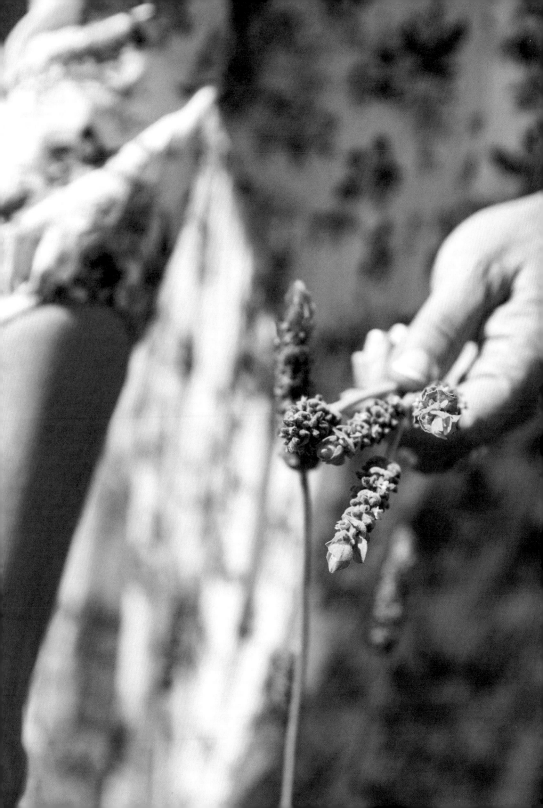

The experience of isolation may vary for everyone; there is no single reason why you may feel isolated. Make sure you reach out and seek support from healthcare professionals, family and friends to help you manage the physical, emotional and social aspects of this condition.

Don't worry, I've got you. I'd love to share some ways to feel less isolated when you're in the midst of a bout or relapse of Long Covid. I've personally done everything on this list and they all help in their own way.

It helps to talk to someone who doesn't know you. If you're okay to go online, you could join a support group – there are many online and in-person support groups for people with Long Covid. Joining a group can help you connect with others who are going through similar experiences.

Social media can be a powerful tool for finding community and support. When used in a thoughtful and intentional way, social media helps you connect with others and share your experiences. Look for hashtags related to Long Covid or join groups focused on chronic illness. Facebook has several good support groups. They can give you a sense of community and allow you to connect with others who are going through similar experiences. You could also follow Long Covid advocacy groups on X or Instagram. These groups provide updates on the latest research and news.

Some people (including myself) find solace in using social media to educate others. By sharing your own experiences and raising awareness about Long Covid, you can help to reduce its stigma and promote understanding. Many doctors and researchers who specialise in Long Covid are active on social media now and they're providing valuable up-to-date information and resources. I recommend following Dr Jill Carnahan MD and Dr Christine Bishara.

> **LEAN ON YOUR LOVED ONES.** You don't have to go through Long Covid alone. Don't be afraid to reach out to your friends and family for support. Share your experiences with them and let them know what you need to feel better. Sometimes just having someone to talk to can make all the difference. Remember, you're not a burden – your loved ones want to help you through this.

CONSIDER THERAPY to help manage difficult emotions and feelings of isolation. Seeking help is a sign of strength, not weakness. A trained therapist or counsellor can support and guide you through the challenges of this condition. They can offer coping strategies and techniques to help you manage symptoms such as anxiety and depression.

GET OUTSIDE. When we're feeling low, it can seem like there's no way out. But something as simple as stepping outside and feeling the sun on your skin can be a small ray of hope. Being out in nature can be so healing, even if it's just for a few minutes each day.

YOU NEED SELF-CARE FOR YOUR OVERALL WELL-BEING. When dealing with Long Covid, you should prioritise self-care activities – these can help to reduce stress and improve your physical and mental health. Don't feel guilty about taking care of yourself. I know I did, but it's necessary. I took long baths with candles and essential oils, practised meditation and even got massages. In the UK, I called a massage therapist to come to the house once a week and it really lit up my week. These activities not only helped me feel better physically but they also gave me a mental break from the constant worry and anxiety. Remember, focusing on self-care is not selfish but a necessary part of your journey towards healing.

Clearing brain fog – out of the haze and into the clear

If you've ever experienced brain fog, you know how frustrating and debilitating it can be. It's like walking through a dense fog – you can't see or think clearly. For people with Long Covid, brain fog can last for weeks or even months. It can make it difficult to focus, remember things or even carry out simple tasks. But there is hope. With some simple tips and techniques, you can clear the fog and start feeling more like yourself again.

Brain fog may include deficits in spatial planning, working memory and executive functioning, difficulty with word retrieval and fluency and poor attention. COVID-19 doesn't just attack your immune system, but your brain too.

If you find yourself putting your shoes in the fridge, you're not alone. According to a systematic review of 81 studies, about one in five people experienced cognitive impairment (commonly known as brain fog) for at least 12 weeks after being diagnosed with COVID-19. For some, the fog just keeps getting thicker, up to 12 months after the initial virus.

✳ CASE STUDY: SEBASTIAN ✳

Sebastian Thaw is a 55-year old male from London, UK. His encounter with Long Covid began during his flight home from a holiday in Greece in August 2022. The subsequent infection left him bedridden for five weeks. Sebastian's Long Covid symptoms, which continue to this day, include debilitating fatigue, brain fog akin to early dementia and recurrent ear infections. The fatigue confined him to his bed for about half his Long Covid journey, significantly impacting his income and financial stability. The brain fog has posed significant challenges to being able to think clearly and manage his daily life effectively.

Prior to Long Covid, Sebastian led an active lifestyle that included strenuous yoga sessions. But his physical fitness has drastically declined; even simple exercises are unfeasible. While his emotional well-being has been stabilised through antidepressant treatment, the unpredictability of and limitations imposed by Long Covid have taken a toll on Sebastian's overall quality of life.

The fluctuating nature of his symptoms makes it difficult for him to plan or engage in regular activities. The lack of tailored medical expertise and support has left him frustrated and bewildered. Sebastian's story highlights Long Covid's profound impact on an individual's physical, mental and emotional well-being.

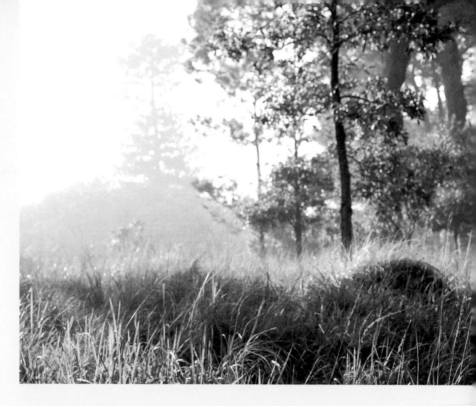

Brain fog can be related to the central nervous system (CNS). The CNS controls and coordinates all the body's functions and processes, including cognitive function, perception and awareness. Brain fog is used to describe a feeling of mental confusion, lack of clarity and difficulty focusing or remembering things. It can be caused by factors that affect the CNS, including stress, lack of sleep, hormonal imbalances and medical conditions such as ME/CFS or fibromyalgia.

A ground-breaking German study revealed that even after COVID-19 clears out of the body, the spike protein may linger in the brain.[44] Shockingly, the researchers found evidence of the spike protein in the brain tissue of deceased animals and humans. Their discovery shows that virus fragments can accumulate in the brain and trigger inflammation, leading to persistent symptoms of Long Covid. The spike protein can linger in the body, making its way into the brain and leading to brain fog and other cognitive issues.

Brain fog from Long Covid is no joke, but that doesn't mean we can't have a laugh while discussing ways to manage it. Alexa, play: 'I can see clearly now the brain fog has gone.'

MY TRIED-AND-TESTED TIPS TO CLEAR THE FOG	
Rest!	That's right, the key to staying sharp and focused is to do nothing. Sounds easy, right? Not exactly. You see, it's not just about sleeping eight hours a night, it's about taking naps, lounging on the couch and basically becoming a professional at doing absolutely nothing. So, let's all pledge to prioritise rest and become masters of the art of laziness. Who's with me?
Exercise	Exercise is good for more than just avoiding dad bods and fitting into skinny jeans. It can clear the cobwebs from your noggin and help you think more clearly. Who knew? Put on those sweatbands, dust off your old Jane Fonda VHS tapes and get ready to sweat out that brain fog. Just don't forget to stretch first!
Healthy eats	Give your brain a boost with some healthy eats. Put down the processed snacks and pick up some brain food, such as fish high in omega-3 fatty acids, leafy greens and colourful fruits and veggies. Your brain will thank you, and who knows? Maybe you'll even remember where you put your keys.
Water	Speaking of food, don't let your brain turn into a dried-up raisin! Staying hydrated will help to combat your muddled brain. Water is your friend, so drink up! If you need to mix things up a bit, try some hydrating fruits like blueberry or cucumber. Just don't go overboard and make it actual 'fruit punch', or you might end up with a whole different kind of fog, nudge nudge, wink wink.
Negative ions	These are electrically charged particles that can have positive effects on cognitive performance, mental capacity and brain function, so they're beneficial if you're experiencing brain fog or cognitive difficulties. As well as their positive effects on cognition, negative ions also have antimicrobial properties. Negative ions can inhibit the growth of bacteria and disrupt their stability, which can help with maintaining a healthy balance of microorganisms in the body. One natural source of negative ions is fulvic humic concentrate, a nutrient and energy booster that aids the body in filtering out bacteria, parasites and fungi.
Cognitive exercises	As someone who holds the Scrabble crown, let me tell you, there's more to life than word games. (Just kidding, there really isn't.) If you want to clear the fog and take back your cognitive prowess, try some mind-bending activities like crossword puzzles, sudoku and even meditation. Give your brain the workout it deserves! If all else fails, just challenge your friends to a game of Scrabble – victory is the ultimate brain boost.

Autonomic dysfunction in Long Covid

We've talked about how your body has an assistant that takes care of all the things you don't even think about, like your heart rate, digestion and temperature control. It's called the autonomic nervous system, or as I like to call it, the 'ANS-droid'! Sometimes, especially in the case of Long Covid, this trusty assistant can go haywire and cause all sorts of trouble.

The ANS acts automatically without requiring conscious effort or awareness, and is responsible for maintaining homeostasis in the body. This means it keeps bodily functions within a normal range and responds to changes in the environment to maintain this balance. The ANS is divided into two branches: the sympathetic and parasympathetic nervous systems.

The sympathetic nervous system (I remember it by saying it's the one you need to feel sorry for) prepares the body for fight-or-flight responses to stress or danger. It increases heart rate, dilates the pupils and inhibits digestion. The parasympathetic nervous system, on the other hand, is responsible for rest-and-digest responses, slowing down the heart rate, constricting the pupils and stimulating digestion. You need a balance between the two for your body to function properly.

Stress activates two main pathways in the body: the pituitary–adrenal axis, which increases the production of stress-regulating hormones, and the ANS. When the ANS doesn't function as it's meant to, this can contribute to Long Covid.

People with Long Covid may experience ANS issues such as dysautonomia, which is a dysfunction of the ANS[45] with symptoms such as rapid heart rate, blood pressure fluctuations, gastrointestinal symptoms, and dizziness or light-headedness upon standing. Some patients with Long Covid may experience POTS, which is having a rapid heart rate and other symptoms upon standing up from a lying or sitting position.

According to Dr David Putrino, the director of rehabilitation innovation at the Mount Sinai Health System in New York, USA, about

80 per cent of patients in his practice meet the criteria for dysautonomia. Other studies have found that about two-thirds of individuals with Long Covid have dysautonomia.

✳ TILT TABLE TEST ✳

A relatively straightforward method to diagnose dysautonomia is by conducting a tilt table test. This test is useful for assessing POTS, one of the most common forms of dysautonomia. During the tilt table test, the patient lies flat on a table. The head of the table is gradually raised to an almost upright position as the patient's heart rate and blood pressure are carefully monitored. Signs of POTS include an abnormal increase in heart rate upon assuming an upright position, along with a worsening of symptoms.

The tilt table test helps healthcare providers to gather valuable diagnostic information and identify if dysautonomia (particularly POTS) is present in patients experiencing Long Covid. This means they can implement appropriate treatment and management strategies to address the specific symptoms and challenges of dysautonomia.

The relationship between COVID-19 and the ANS is complicated. On one hand, the virus can induce sympathetic activation, leading to a cytokine storm and pro-inflammatory responses. On the other hand, stimulation of the vagus nerve can result in anti-inflammatory responses, opening up potential therapeutic targets in the ANS. But that's not all. Another theory is that COVID-19 may directly mediate autonomic dysfunction. It's possible that some or all of these mechanisms may overlap.

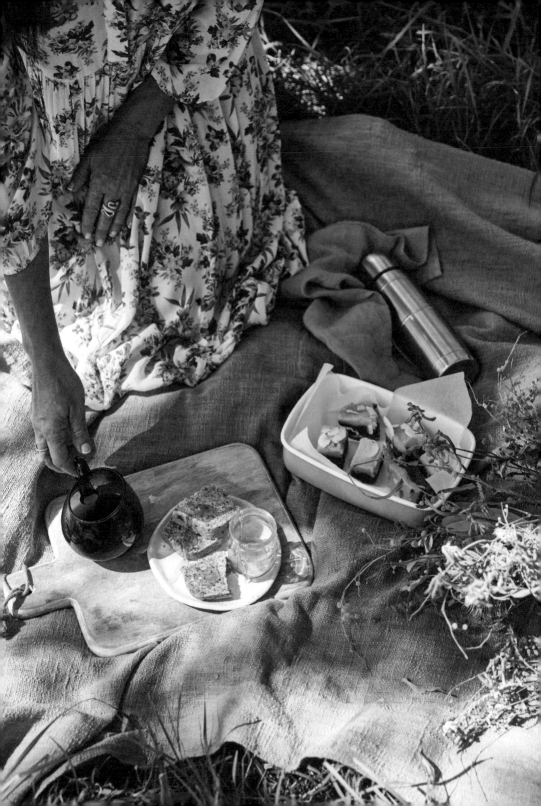

Postural orthostatic tachycardia syndrome

POTS is a type of dysautonomia, or ANS dysfunction, that is characterised by an abnormal increase in heart rate upon standing. POTS is a form of orthostatic intolerance, which means that symptoms are triggered by changes in posture, particularly when moving from lying down or sitting to standing.

Along with an increased heart rate, POTS can cause symptoms such as dizziness, light-headedness, fainting and fatigue. You know that feeling when you're lightheaded after standing up too fast? It's like your heart decides to go on a joyride when you stand up, racing up to 120 beats per minute within 10 minutes. And as if that's not enough, you also experience a dizzy spell that can make you feel like you're auditioning for a role in a zombie movie. But wait, there's more! POTS comes with a range of delightful symptoms such as brain fog, headaches, fatigue and sleep disturbances too.

Current research suggests that POTS in Long Covid patients may be related to a combination of factors. One possible mechanism is the persistent inflammation in the body, a key feature of Long Covid. This inflammation may damage the ANS, which can lead to dysautonomia and POTS. Long Covid may also be associated with endothelial dysfunction, which can affect blood vessel function and contribute to POTS symptoms. Some forms of POTS have been associated with MCAS.[46]

Dealing with POTS can be challenging and frustrating, but resources and strategies are available to help you manage symptoms and improve your quality of life. If Long Covid has you feeling like a human slinky, here are some helpful tips:

INCREASE YOUR FLUID AND SALT INTAKE. Drinking plenty of fluids and getting enough salt can help to raise your blood volume, which may improve symptoms.

WEAR COMPRESSION STOCKINGS. Compression stockings help to improve blood flow and may help alleviate symptoms such as light-headedness or fainting.

EXERCISE REGULARLY. Low-impact exercises such as walking or swimming may improve your blood flow and cardiovascular function, which can help to alleviate symptoms of POTS. Make sure you work with a healthcare provider to develop an exercise program that is safe and appropriate for you.

AVOID TRIGGERS. Certain foods, medications and activities may trigger POTS. Identifying and avoiding these triggers may help improve your symptoms. When I had POTS episodes, I found that monosodium glutamate (MSG, a common food additive) caused symptoms as well as processed foods with additives and too much sugar. Caffeine was a big one for me, even chai tea sadly, so I gave that up while I was recovering. Some individuals with POTS may be sensitive to dairy products, which can cause inflammation and exacerbate their symptoms. For me, dairy wasn't a problem.

MANAGE YOUR STRESS. Stress can exacerbate symptoms of POTS in several ways. When you experience stress, your body releases stress hormones such as cortisol and adrenaline, which cause the heart rate and blood pressure to increase. With POTS, this can trigger symptoms such as dizziness, light-headedness and fainting. Practices such as meditation, deep breathing exercises or yoga may help to reduce stress and improve symptoms.

CONSIDER MEDICATIONS OR SUPPLEMENTS. Your GP may prescribe medications such as beta blockers, fludrocortisone and midodrine to help alleviate symptoms of POTS. If you prefer a holistic route, which I took, natural supplements helped me to manage my symptoms.

NATURAL SUPPLEMENTS TO HELP POTS	
Salt	Increasing your salt intake can help increase blood volume and improve symptoms of POTS. Make sure you work with a healthcare provider to determine the appropriate amount of salt for you.
Magnesium	This can help to improve blood flow and reduce symptoms such as palpitations and chest pain.
Coenzyme Q10	This antioxidant may help to improve heart function and reduce symptoms of POTS.
Vitamin D	Low levels of vitamin D have been linked to POTS symptoms, so supplementing with vitamin D may help improve symptoms.
B-complex vitamins	These vitamins can help to improve energy levels and reduce fatigue, which are common symptoms of POTS.

Making these changes and exercising regularly can help you manage symptoms. In some cases, other therapies such as physiotherapy or acupuncture may be useful. Psychological interventions such as cognitive-behavioural therapy have shown promise in managing symptoms such as anxiety and depression. Other emerging treatments to explore are non-medication approaches, IV saline infusions, immune-modulating therapies and transcranial magnetic stimulation.

Post-exertional malaise

A common symptom of POTS is post-exertional malaise (PEM). A 2021 study reported that almost three-quarters of people with Long Covid symptoms lasting at least seven months experienced PEM.

With PEM, you experience a worsening of symptoms after physical or mental activity, which can be a significant challenge when managing Long Covid. I had terrible PEM after COVID-19. It was a feeling of intense fatigue and exhaustion that set in after even minimal physical or mental exertion. It's very similar to what I experienced when I had chronic fatigue.

PEM is a distinct phenomenon that goes beyond mere feelings of tiredness. Dr Putrino emphasises the difference between PEM and fatigue, noting that he observes it in about 90 per cent of patients visiting his Long Covid clinic.

PEM can be a constant source of frustration, anxiety and despair because all you want to do is live a normal life, but you find yourself to be unable to work, exercise, socialise or pursue your passions. It's like your body is betraying you, like every step you take, every thought you have, is draining you of precious energy.

PEM can cause fatigue, brain fog, dizziness and muscle weakness, which worsen after physical or mental exertion. This usually occurs a day or two after the activity, but it can last for days and sometimes weeks after the initial exertion. If you have POTS, it needs careful management to minimise its impact on your daily life.

Dysautonomia

Dr Groysman has been treating Long Covid patients for three years. I asked him whether he had any advice for treating patients with dysautonomia, which he considered was the cause of other symptoms such as dizziness, fatigue, brain fog, difficulty sleeping and digestive issues.

He advised it was important to treat the cause, which is often the dysautonomia. He recommends several successful treatment options. Reduce your stress levels – physical and mental stress are linked to dysautonomia and can make symptoms worse. He also suggested breathing exercises, yoga or anything that relaxes the patient. He added, 'External vagus nerve stimulation can help reduce the severity as well as reducing stress in your life. There are breathing exercises and breath work that can help reduce the severity of your symptoms. There has been recent evidence that metformin, an oral medicine taken for diabetes mellitus, especially if taken early in COVID-19 infection, can help reduce the risk of Long Covid by 42 per cent. Knowing your risk is also helpful. Recent studies have shown that women are more at risk than men. Being overweight, smoking, and having other autoimmune conditions can also predispose to getting Long Covid.[47] Also older adults are more at risk than children.'

In the context of Long Covid, dysautonomia may be a contributing factor to persistent symptoms such as PEM and orthostatic intolerance.

So, while dysautonomia may not be the sole cause of these symptoms, it can play a significant role in their development and persistence.

Several lifestyle modifications may help to improve dysautonomia symptoms, including wearing compression stockings and keeping your stress levels down. I have some great breathing exercises coming up that you can try (see page 99). A simple change is ensuring you stay hydrated. Certain foods, medications and activities may trigger dysautonomia. Identifying and avoiding these triggers may help improve your symptoms.

SOME COMMON TRIGGERS OF DYSAUTONOMIA	
High-carbohydrate or high-sugar foods	These foods can cause blood sugar spikes and drops, which can trigger symptoms.
Caffeine	Caffeine can stimulate the nervous system and increase heart rate and blood pressure, which can exacerbate symptoms.
Alcohol	Alcohol can also stimulate the nervous system and increase heart rate and blood pressure.
Processed foods and artificial sweeteners	These foods can contain additives and preservatives that may trigger symptoms in some individuals.
Certain medications	Some medications, including blood-pressure medications, diuretics and antidepressants, can have side effects that exacerbate symptoms.
Prolonged standing or sitting	Remaining in the same position for long periods of time can lead to blood pooling in the legs and exacerbate symptoms.

Identifying and avoiding triggers may take some trial and error, because they can vary among individuals.

Heat and Long Covid

Heat can be a cruel and unforgiving adversary for people with Long Covid. I know all too well how heat can trigger a cascade of symptoms and inflammation in my body, leaving me feeling weak and helpless.

Because Long Covid is characterised by dysautonomia, it can manifest as light-headedness and heart palpitations or even an intolerance to heat.

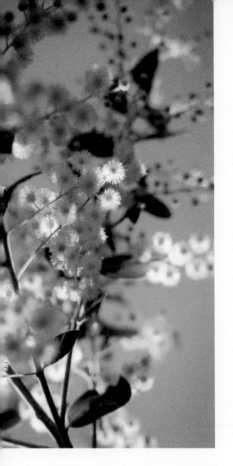

I live at the beach. During Long Covid, even a few minutes in the sun felt like an eternity, as my body struggled to regulate its core temperature and maintain a sense of balance. I remember walking down to the seashore. It was a warm day, the sun was shining and the sea breeze was gently prickling my skin. It felt good to be outside in its refreshing embrace. But as I sat down on the shore, I soon realised that the heat was too much for me to bear. Despite my best intentions, I quickly overheated, and my body was not happy. My heart raced, my head spun and I knew I had to leave before things got worse. As I walked home, defeated and exhausted, my body was aching and my spirit broken. I had just overheated – I knew that I'd end up flaking out for the rest of the day.

When the body is exposed to high temperatures, it can trigger an immune response that can cause inflammation. Because inflammation contributes to Long Covid symptoms, exposure to heat may exacerbate inflammation and thus make symptoms worse.

Heat can also contribute to dehydration, which can worsen symptoms of Long Covid. Dehydration can cause fatigue and brain fog, which can make it more difficult to manage symptoms. I found that I'd bounce back quicker when I drank plenty of water. It's important to replenish your fluids regularly.

You need to keep cool when dealing with Long Covid. You can achieve this by keeping your living space cool with air conditioning or fans, and not going outside during the hottest parts of the day. If you do need to go outside, consider wearing lightweight, breathable clothing and a hat to shield yourself from the sun. These small adjustments can make a big difference in your well-being. If you need to be in a warm environment, you can find cooling products to help improve your quality of life. Cooling vests, neck wraps and towels are just a few examples of products that work by absorbing moisture and evaporating sweat, helping to regulate your body temperature and keep you cool. I found wearing breathable fabrics and linen helped and I always wore a hat.

Downregulate the nervous system

We know that Long Covid can be associated with dysregulation of the ANS. Studies also show decreased PNS activity and increased sympathetic nervous system (SNS) activity.[48] This may lead to fatigue, brain fog and exercise intolerance, as well as other physical and psychological symptoms.

Downregulating the ANS means reducing the activity of the SNS, which prepares the body for stress or danger. Chronic activation of the SNS can lead to negative health outcomes, including chronic stress, anxiety and inflammation. By downregulating the ANS, your body can achieve a state of relaxation and support its natural healing processes.

Mind–body techniques, such as mindfulness meditation and deep breathing exercises, help to regulate the ANS and reduce stress and anxiety.

The nervous system sometimes feels like an overachiever who's gone into overdrive, but you can put it back in its place by downregulating. Benefits include reduced stress – a real lifesaver in today's world. Chronic stress is a one-way ticket to health problems from heart disease to tummy troubles and mental health woes. So, if you want to live your best life, it's time to give your nervous system a chill pill.

Next on the list is improved sleep. You know the drill – stress and anxiety can mess with your sleep patterns, leaving you feeling groggy and irritable. But fear not, downregulating can help you catch those zzz's like a pro.

Let's not forget about inflammation – the bane of many a chronic condition including Long Covid. Chronic stress can cause inflammation in the body, leading to all sorts of health issues, but with downregulating, you can calm down the inflammation. Last but not least, downregulating leads to improved immune function. When stress is chronic, your immune system is weakened, making you more susceptible to all sorts of bugs.

WAYS TO DOWNREGULATE OR CALM THE NERVOUS SYSTEM	
Deep breathing	Slow, deep breathing activates the parasympathetic nervous system, which helps to calm the body and reduce stress.
Mindfulness meditation	Practising mindfulness meditation can help to reduce anxiety and activate the parasympathetic nervous system.
Progressive muscle relaxation	This technique involves tensing then relaxing different muscle groups in the body, which can help to release tension and promote relaxation.
Yoga	Practising yoga can reduce stress and tension in the body, helping to downregulate the nervous system.
Exercise	Regular exercise can reduce stress and anxiety and promote overall well-being.
Spending time in nature	This can help to reduce stress and promote relaxation, downregulating the nervous system.
Engaging in enjoyable activities	Doing activities that you enjoy, such as reading a book, listening to music or spending time with friends and family, can help with stress reduction and relaxation.

Because we're all different, it's good to experiment with different techniques to find what works best for you. If you are struggling with chronic stress or anxiety, seek the support of a mental health professional who can provide you with guidance and support. Techniques could include counselling, yoga, journalling, meditation, guided imagery and breathing exercises. The breathing exercises not only help with anxiety and stress, but can also improve the breathlessness post-COVID-19 patients often feel, particularly those with pulmonary fibrosis.

Become aware of what contributes to your fight, flight or freeze responses – past trauma and triggers, overwhelm, relationships, environment, finances, security, career, caffeine, sugar and nutritional deficiencies, to name a few.

Create touch points of regulation. This could be a candle, prayer, cup of tea, time in nature or connecting with a friend – simple tools to access at any given moment.

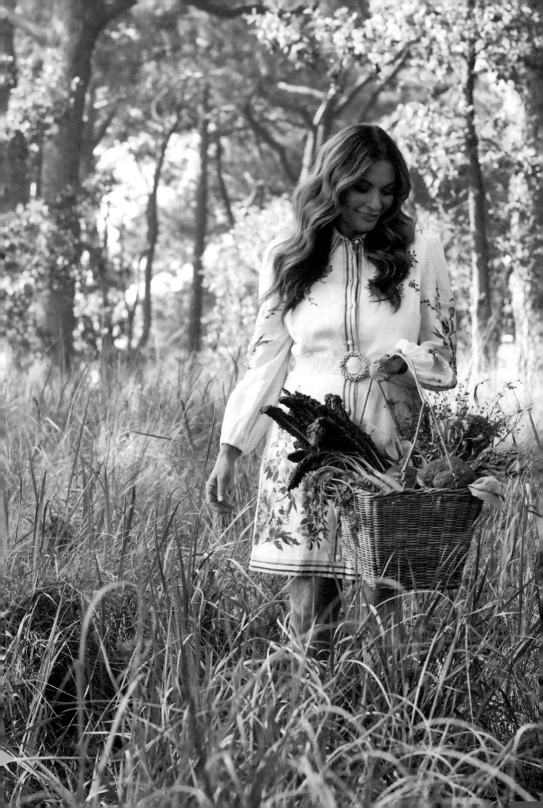

Fatigue

Don't feel guilty about embracing the pyjama lifestyle: with Long Covid comes a truckload of fatigue, so why not embrace loungewear? Who needs pants with buttons when you can wear comfy casuals all day long? Just make sure to switch your daytime jarmies for your night-time PJs before bed.

Fatigue can be different for everyone. For some it's a feeling of tiredness, weakness or exhaustion that can be physical, mental or both. Fatigue can be caused by factors such as lack of sleep, physical exertion, illness, stress and mental health conditions such as depression or anxiety. It can manifest in different ways, including feeling sleepy or drowsy, having difficulty concentrating, feeling weak or achy, or experiencing low energy or motivation. It can also be temporary (lasting for a short period) or chronic (persisting for weeks or months). Long Covid patients with fatigue often describe it as an ongoing, overwhelming tiredness that interferes with their daily activities and quality of life.

The links between Long Covid and fatigue are related to the ongoing inflammation and immune system dysregulation that can occur after a COVID-19 infection. The virus may also directly affect the CNS or damage the nervous system, leading to persistent fatigue.

We know that the virus can damage the cardiovascular system and lungs, affecting oxygen delivery to the body's tissues and contributing to feelings of fatigue. Some people with Long Covid experience neurological symptoms such as brain fog, which contributes to their feelings of fatigue and difficulty concentrating.

According to one study, almost half of the 41 Long Covid patients evaluated met the diagnostic criteria for ME/CFS.[49] This post-viral syndrome can leave at least a quarter of sufferers bed- or house-bound for extended periods, which highlights the challenges faced by people living with Long Covid and the potential long-term consequences of this condition.

The Sagol Center for Hyperbaric Medicine and Research in Israel has developed a promising therapy for brain fog and exhaustion. Long Covid patients undergo daily 90-minute sessions in a hyperbaric oxygen chamber, which promotes the growth of mitochondria, the power source of cells.

This leads to improved energy metabolism and function. Shai Efrati, a professor of neuroscience at Tel Aviv University, led a two-month study involving hyperbaric treatments for 73 Long Covid patients, showing that their overall condition improved. Novel treatments like this offer hope for individuals struggling with the debilitating symptoms of Long Covid.

Long Covid and myalgic encephalomyelitis/chronic fatigue syndrome

So how is Long Covid fatigue similar to chronic fatigue?

For more than a century, post-viral syndromes have been observed following infections with viruses such as HIV and influenza. One virus, Epstein–Barr, which is responsible for mononucleosis (glandular fever), has been linked to a condition known as myalgic encephalomyelitis/chronic fatigue syndrome (ME/CFS). The term 'myalgic encephalomyelitis' refers to the muscle pain and inflammation that can occur in people with ME/CFS, while 'chronic fatigue syndrome' describes the persistent fatigue that is a hallmark of the condition. The inclusion of both terms acknowledges the complexity and severity of this illness.

ME/CFS is estimated to impact about 250,000 people in Australia and more than 1.5 million people in the USA. Long Covid shares similarities with ME/CFS, including immune system dysregulation, fatigue and cognitive dysfunction. Healthcare providers are increasingly observing and treating the conditions accordingly, says William Pittman, a physician at UCLA Health in Los Angeles.

Researchers are investigating whether ME/CFS, like certain cases of Long Covid, may have an autoimmune component, in which autoantibodies perpetuate immune system activation. Autoantibodies are antibodies that target and attack the body's own cells and tissues, leading to inflammation and tissue damage. In the case of ME/CFS, autoantibodies could be triggering the immune system to remain in a state of heightened activity, leading to the condition's characteristic symptoms of fatigue, cognitive dysfunction and immune system dysregulation.

COMMON SYMPTOMS OF ME/CFS	
Persistent and unexplained fatigue	Often described as feeling 'flu-like', this fatigue is not relieved by rest.
Post-exertional malaise	Physical or mental activity can worsen symptoms, leading to a 'crash' or worsening of fatigue that can last for days or even weeks.
Cognitive impairment	This includes difficulty concentrating, memory problems or brain fog.
Sleep disturbances	Sleep may be disrupted, and individuals with ME/CFS may experience unrefreshing sleep or insomnia.
Muscle pain and weakness	Muscle pain, weakness and joint pain are common in ME/CFS.
Headaches	People with ME/CFS describe these as tension-type headaches or migraines.
Digestive problems	Symptoms include nausea, bloating and abdominal pain.

Given the similarities between the symptoms of ME/CFS and Long Covid, researchers are exploring the potential overlap between these conditions. One hypothesis is that Long Covid may be a form of ME/CFS triggered by SARS-CoV-2 infection. This has important implications for the diagnosis and treatment of Long Covid, because ME/CFS is a complex and difficult-to-treat condition that requires a multi-disciplinary approach.

One study published in *BMC Medicine* examined the prevalence of ME/CFS-like symptoms among individuals who had recovered from COVID-19, finding that 45.2 per cent of participants reported ME/CFS-like symptoms such as fatigue, cognitive impairment and sleep disturbances. Individuals with more severe initial COVID-19 symptoms were also more likely to develop ME/CFS-like symptoms. [50]

About 75 per cent of people with ME/CFS experience an infection-like episode before the onset of their illness, suggesting that viral, bacterial or other infections may trigger or contribute to the development of ME/CFS in some individuals.

Some people who develop post-infectious autoimmune syndromes (PAISs) meet the diagnostic criteria for ME/CFS. For example, patients who develop PAISs such as POTS or autoimmune encephalitis may experience fatigue, cognitive problems and muscle pain, symptoms that overlap with ME/CFS. This suggests that ME/CFS may be a type of PAIS triggered by infections.

Bacteria, viruses and parasites have all been linked to the development of PAIS, yet the association between acute infectious diseases and chronic disability remains poorly understood and understudied, leading to inadequate recognition and treatment.

Long Covid and ME/CFS share several key features, including fatigue, muscle pain, brain fog and mitochondrial dysfunction. The nonspecific nature of these symptoms, however, can make it difficult for healthcare professionals to diagnose these conditions, leading to delayed or missed diagnoses. We need increased awareness, research and improved diagnostic tools and criteria to help identify and treat these complex and debilitating conditions.

Researchers are currently trying to disentangle the common features of Long Covid and ME/CFS from their potential causes, including immune system dysregulation, blood clots and viral reactivation and persistence. While the complexity of these conditions means it's challenging to identify the best therapy for each patient, some doctors and researchers suggest using existing treatment protocols for ME/CFS. If you've had a reactivation of ME/CFS, I include a protocol with nutritional supplements that has benefited patients with ME/CFS, myself included (see pages 162–4).

Lorrie Rivers, who developed ME/CFS during college, draws parallels between it and Long Covid. She experienced severe symptoms and was bedridden, relying on her father for assistance. At that time, she was unaware of the importance of pacing when managing the condition. It took her 8–10 years to regain her previous level of functioning. Lorrie has since become an ME/CFS coach who has been helping others for more than 20 years at livingfrominspiration.com.

In May 2020, after contracting COVID-19, Lorrie initially improved but later experienced a decline. She recognised a return of her ME/CFS

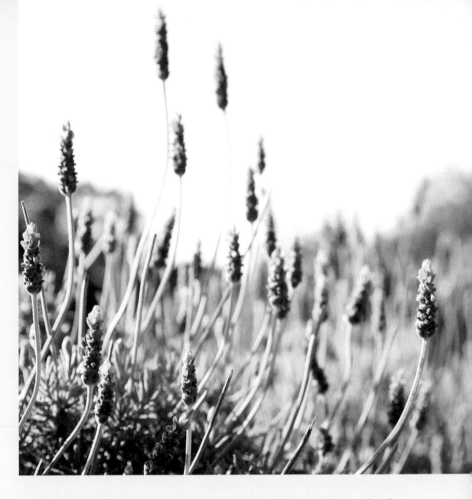

symptoms. Feeling overwhelmed and thinking of the challenges ahead, her coaching practices kicked in, allowing her to regain hope and believe in her ability to overcome the condition once more.

Lorrie's understanding, based on her work with clients and personal experience, is that everyone's Long Covid experience is unique. Her specific symptoms included profound fatigue, brain fog, inner trembling and nervous system dysregulation. She believes that the root cause of chronic illness lies in dysbiosis within the body, which can be triggered by infections.

Her approach addresses these underlying infections, including the potential reactivation of viruses like EBV and herpes. Using the analogy of a house infested with termites, Lorrie explains that when our bodies are compromised and a significant stressor like COVID-19 (with its spike protein) enters, it can further destabilise the system. In the case of Long Covid, she emphasises the importance of addressing the spike protein and underlying infections to facilitate recovery. Immune-modulating medications may also benefit: studies show that low-dose naltrexone (LDN) is safe to use in patients with Long Covid. In a recent 11-month study of patients with Long Covid, LDN reduced their symptoms at two months, as well as their well-being in six of seven parameters.[51]

Five ways to manage Long Covid fatigue

Long Covid is a complex and unpredictable condition that can cause debilitating fatigue that can last for months and even years. Coping with this level of fatigue can be daunting, especially when it interferes with your daily activities and quality of life. It can impact family, relationships, work and your own mental health.

Here, we'll explore five effective strategies for managing Long Covid fatigue. These techniques will help you feel more in control of your symptoms and improve your overall well-being. From getting into a flow state to finding deep rest, each strategy offers a unique approach to coping with Long Covid fatigue. By incorporating these techniques into your routine, you'll better manage your symptoms and find greater relief from Long Covid.

1. Getting into a flow state

While dealing with Long Covid fatigue can be enormously challenging, one technique that may help you be more productive is getting into a flow state. This is a mental state of productivity and focus, which seems so unattainable when you're dealing with chronic fatigue. It's like trying to run a marathon wearing a weighted blanket while your brain is stuck in molasses. But don't worry, my fellow long-hauler, I have some easy and doable tips on how to get into the flow state even when your energy is running on empty.

Just to clear things up, let's redefine the flow state as the 'slow state'. You may need to take things at a slower pace than others, and that's perfectly okay. Embrace it. It's a luxurious, leisurely stroll rather than a sprint. You can still get things done, but without the added pressure of racing against the clock.

To help you get into a flow state, create an environment that supports your energy levels – this is going to be different for everyone. It might mean taking frequent breaks from what you're doing, setting up a comfortable area for tasks or even using a standing desk if you're back to working (standing desks help to combat brain fog).

Rewind the clock and think back to a time when you've felt serene. A mood where time seems to pass more slowly, and you don't feel pressed for time. I like to call it the 'gentle flow state'; this mental state will let you fully focus on the activity at hand without feeling rushed or under pressure.

Being productive in the flow state involves being present in the moment and appreciating the journey, rather than hurrying, working harder or pushing yourself to complete a task. Even regular routine duties can turn into enjoyable activities because you can appreciate their subtleties and particulars. In your mind picture serenely drifting down a river without a concern in the world.

Being in the flow state means being kind to yourself. Instead of attempting to force anything, give yourself permission to immerse yourself in what you're doing. The best part is that you finish feeling renewed and invigorated, rather than worn out and even more fatigued. When starting out, breathe deeply, do some gentle stretches or yoga or simply sit outside to prepare yourself for getting into flow. You're recharging your batteries to help you get into a more relaxed, focused state of mind, leading you to a more conscious and satisfying way of functioning.

You know you've entered the zone when you lose track of time, forget to check your phone and find yourself impervious to distractions (with the possible exception of the occasional cute animal video because, let's face it, they're hard to resist). The ultimate benefit of being in flow is the joy of a task well done, which is like a delicious piece of pie for your brain.

The flow state is like an ideal state between procrastination and workaholism. At that beautiful moment, your brain chooses to connect with the task at hand and you don't feel pressured to complete it. A key to getting into this state is finding the right level of challenge – not too easy, but not too hard either. We call this the 'Goldilocks zone' of difficulty, which is different for everyone.

Here are some of my tips for getting into a flow state when you've got Long Covid but need to get things done. I've incorporated them into my own healing journey and they've been immeasurably helpful:

PICK A TASK THAT IS LEVEL TWO DIFFICULT BUT STILL DOABLE. Flow is more likely to happen when you're working on something that is difficult enough to demand all your attention but not so hard that you feel overwhelmed or frustrated. For example, you might have a pile of laundry that needs washing – it's not the most exciting task, but it requires a certain level of focus and attention to detail. The beauty of doing laundry (or any task that's level two difficult but doable) is that it allows your brain to focus on the task without getting bogged down by too much complexity or confusion. You can create a sense of order and accomplishment by completing each step of the process, from separating the colours to folding and putting away the clean clothes. And the best part? Once you've finished the task, you'll have a tangible sense of achievement – a pile of fresh, clean laundry that's ready to be worn and enjoyed.

ESTABLISH SMALL GOALS. Begin with a task that is small and achievable, such as reading a chapter of a book or writing for 10 minutes. Small goals are more manageable and less overwhelming than larger goals, and can help you build momentum towards bigger achievements. Break them down: take a larger goal and break it down into smaller, more manageable chunks. For example, if your goal is to clean your entire house, break it down into smaller tasks such as cleaning one room per day or even just wiping down the kitchen counters. When you are early in your recovery, that can be all you can manage some days.

MINIMISE DISTRACTIONS. You need to do some work, but your mind is jumping all over the place. Picture this: you're settling in to get some work done. You're feeling demotivated but need to tackle one or two things on your to-do list. But then your phone buzzes with a notification, your email inbox pings with a new message, and before you know it, you're deep in a social media rabbit hole. Reduce those interruptions and minimise distractions as much as possible, especially if you have chronic fatigue and over-sensitisation (many people with Long Covid have this). I like to set up a space in a separate room. The first thing I do is disable notifications on my phone and computer. It's amazing how much of a difference it can make – not having those constant buzzes and beeps vying for your attention. When I'm feeling really distracted, I put my phone in another room or turn it off altogether. Next, I close any unnecessary computer tabs and programs. This lets me focus better on the task at hand, so I'm fully engaged in the activity, focusing my attention solely on that task.

TAKE BREAKS. Taking brief rest periods will let you re-energise and prevent burnout. The best approach for taking a break will depend on your personal preferences and energy levels. Some people find that going for a gentle stroll in the fresh air can be a refreshing break from sedentary activities. Others may prefer gentle stretching or yoga poses to loosen up their stiff muscles and improve circulation. Still others may enjoy activities that offer mental stimulation, such as reading, meditating or listening to calming music. When you're feeling fatigued, taking a brief rest period can help you re-energise and recharge, both physically and mentally.

PUT IN FREQUENT PRACTICE. Flow is a condition you can learn. Make it a habit to regularly do things that need your undivided attention and focus. Practising flow doesn't mean pushing yourself beyond your limits or ignoring your body's needs. Instead, it's about finding the right level of challenge that lets you fully engage in a task and experience a sense of accomplishment.

BE KIND TO YOURSELF. Dealing with Long Covid fatigue is challenging, and it's okay if you can't work for extended periods of time. Be gentle with yourself and take things at your own pace to manage this condition and allow your body to heal.

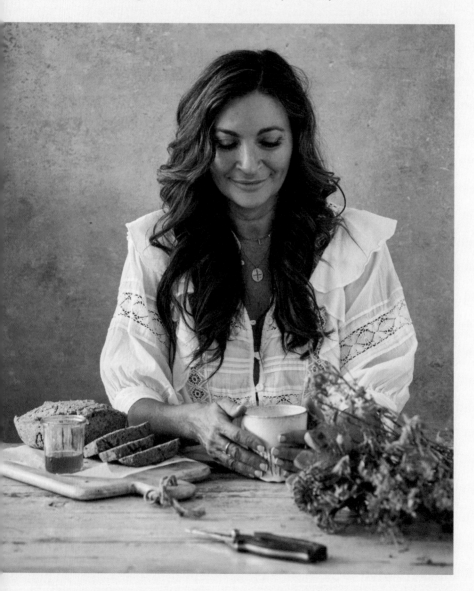

When you're feeling fatigued, you may be tempted to push yourself to get things done, but this can lead to burnout and make your symptoms worse. Instead, try to be patient and compassionate with yourself. Listen to your body and take breaks when you need to, even if it means slowing down your work pace or taking longer to complete tasks.

The flow state is a deeply personal experience: what works for one person may not work for another. Experiment with different techniques to find what works best for you. By getting into a flow state, you may discover you can work more efficiently and with less stress, which can help you manage your Long Covid fatigue more effectively. Don't forget to check in with yourself, listen to your body's cues and take breaks because overexertion can exacerbate your fatigue symptoms.

2. Acupuncture

In this ancient Chinese therapy, tiny needles are inserted into specific points on the body. It can help to reduce inflammation, boost the immune system, and promote overall health and well-being.

Acupuncture may be helpful for people with Long Covid.[52] A study published in the *Journal of Medical Acupuncture* investigated the potential benefits of acupuncture for Long Covid. It involved 11 participants who were experiencing symptoms such as fatigue, shortness of breath and brain fog, who received acupuncture treatments twice a week for four weeks. The participants reported significant improvements in their symptoms after receiving acupuncture treatments, specifically fatigue, shortness of breath and overall quality of life. They also reported improvements in their anxiety and depression symptoms.

Acupuncture, the superhero we need in the fight against Long Covid fatigue, has some serious powers up its sleeve! Its pain-relieving abilities can vanquish those pesky muscle and joint aches, while its stress- and anxiety-reducing capabilities can provide much-needed calm. Acupuncture's calming effects can help you find some much-needed peace in the midst of the chaos.

Acupuncture has immune-modulating effects, which means it can help to regulate the immune system, promoting healing and recovery. By modulating the immune system, acupuncture may help to calm down inflammation and promote overall wellness – a benefit for people with Long Covid!

By improving blood flow and circulation, acupuncture can help to deliver oxygen and nutrients to tissues affected by Long Covid, which can promote healing and reduce inflammation. Improved circulation can also help the body eliminate waste and toxins, further supporting the healing process.

If Long Covid has disrupted your sleep, let acupuncture come to the rescue. Its ability to improve sleep quality makes it a valuable ally for anyone struggling with sleep disruptions. By promoting relaxation and reducing stress, acupuncture can help ease you into a more restful state. And when you're getting the rest you need, your body is better equipped to fight off the lingering effects of the virus.

3. Pacing

Pacing is the art of taking things at a steady and sustainable pace. This is a helpful strategy for managing chronic illness or conditions characterised by fatigue or pain, such as fibromyalgia, ME/CFS and Long Covid. Pacing involves carefully balancing activity and rest to conserve energy and avoid exacerbating symptoms. Instead of sprinting through your day and crashing at the finish line, pacing helps you break down your tasks into manageable chunks and take regular breaks to recharge.

Pacing is based on the idea that people with chronic illnesses have a limited amount of energy available to them each day, so they must carefully manage their activities to avoid running out of energy and experiencing symptom flare-ups. It's like a game of 'Long Covid survivor' – if you pace yourself, you'll be the last one standing!

For example, you might pace your activities by doing a few minutes of light exercise, such as gentle yoga or stretching, followed by a period of rest, then gradually increase the duration and intensity of exercise over time. You might also plan rest breaks throughout the day and prioritise activities that promote relaxation and well-being, such as meditation or taking a warm bath.

When I employed pacing by breaking my daily activities into smaller, manageable tasks and taking regular breaks to prevent overexertion and exhaustion, the next day my fatigue and brain fog would feel better. If I pushed through, however, I often felt worse the next day, which made my symptoms even more debilitating. I learned to be gentle with myself and listen to my body's cues. In the first few months I could hardly do anything at all, but I leaned into it and didn't beat myself up. When I did very slowly regain energy, I made sure I only did small things each day and didn't overdo it.

For example, I would start my day with a small task like making breakfast or checking emails then take a short break to rest or do something relaxing. Doing gentle exercises like yoga or stretching helped me to maintain my energy levels and avoid feeling too fatigued. It was a balance between no exercise at all, which can make us feel tired, and too much exercise, which also leaves us feeling fatigued.

At times it was challenging to pace myself, because I felt like I wasn't accomplishing as much as I wanted to. But I reminded myself that taking care of my health was my top priority; it was okay to take things slow. With time, pacing became a natural part of my daily routine and helped me manage my Long Covid symptoms more effectively.

To implement pacing, identify your energy limits and prioritise your daily tasks. Divide your tasks into smaller, manageable portions. Remember to take regular breaks, rest when you need and avoid pushing yourself beyond your limits. If you need to weed the garden, for instance, break up the task into smaller parts, such as weeding one bed at a time. Take breaks in between each task to rest and recharge your energy. You can also use tools and equipment to make tasks easier and less tiring.

Keep track of symptoms and adjust your activities accordingly, so you can avoid pushing yourself too far and triggering a flare-up. And don't forget to prioritise self-care. Activities that promote relaxation and well-being, such as meditation, gentle yoga or a soothing bath, can be a valuable part of your pacing routine.

By using pacing, you can manage your Long Covid symptoms and still accomplish your daily tasks. Be patient with yourself and don't push yourself too hard. Listen to your body, rest when needed and adjust your pacing to find what works best for you.

✳ WHY PACE IT OUT? ✳

✦ Pacing can help to reduce symptom flare-ups and their frequency and severity.

✦ Conserve energy. Avoid 'boom-and-bust' cycles, where you push yourself too hard on good days then crash when you overdo it.

✦ Improve endurance. By gradually increasing your activity levels over time, you can build endurance and strength.

✦ Reduce stress. By minimising the stress and anxiety associated with symptom flare-ups and overexertion, pacing can help improve your overall well-being.

✦ Set realistic goals. It's better to start small and gradually increase your activity levels over time than to jump in with both feet and risk overexertion.

✦ If you want to try pacing as a way to manage Long Covid symptoms (which if you only do one thing in this book, I highly recommend), then try these 20 ways to do it:

1. Break up tasks into smaller, manageable steps.
2. Prioritise rest breaks throughout the day.
3. Use a timer or alarm to remind you to take breaks.
4. Set yourself realistic goals and expectations.
5. Use energy-saving techniques, such as sitting instead of standing where possible.
6. Delegate tasks to others if you can.
7. Use adaptive equipment, such as a wheelchair or mobility aid, if necessary.
8. Plan out your day in advance to avoid overexertion.
9. Incorporate gentle stretching or low-impact exercise into your daily routine.
10. Practise mindfulness and meditation to reduce stress.
11. Avoid multitasking – focus on one task at a time.
12. Keep a diary or journal to track your symptoms and energy levels.
13. Get enough sleep and prioritise a consistent sleep schedule.
14. Stay hydrated and eat a balanced, nutritious, low-histamine diet.
15. Avoid overstimulation from technology and screens.
16. Don't overexert yourself during physical activities, such as exercise or housework.
17. Take frequent breaks during prolonged periods of sitting or standing.
18. Use relaxation techniques such as deep breathing or progressive muscle relaxation.
19. Use positive self-talk and affirmations to keep motivated.
20. Don't push yourself beyond your limits; listen to your body's signals to rest and recover.

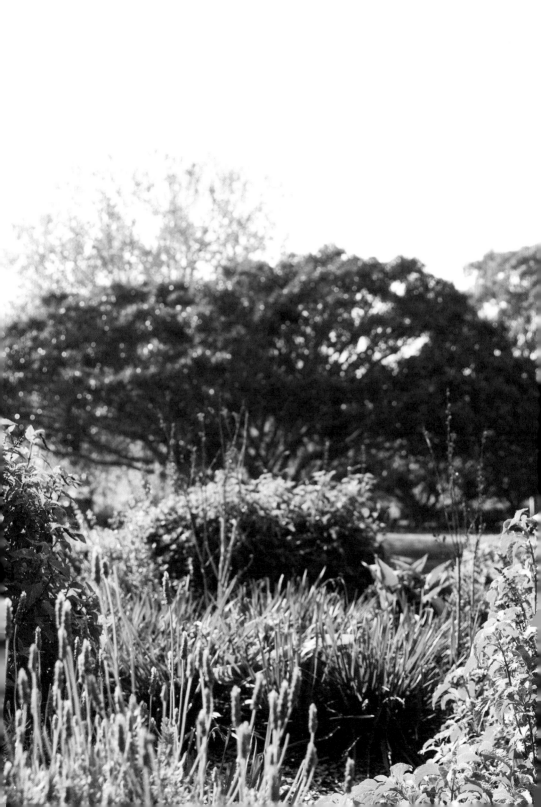

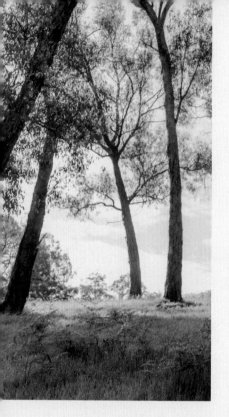

4. Mindfulness

Another strategy that I employed for fatigue was mindfulness. Even just a few minutes of mindfulness each day could make a big difference in how I felt. I practise Vedic meditation, which takes 22 minutes each day. This helps me to stay present and focus on the current moment, rather than worrying about the future or dwelling on the past. I found that meditating reduced my stress levels and improved my overall sense of well-being, which helped to alleviate my fatigue symptoms. I also made a conscious effort to incorporate mindfulness into my daily activities, such as when walking or eating, which helped me to stay present and connected to my body.

Here are some tips to get started:

FIND A QUIET PLACE TO SIT OR EVEN LIE DOWN. Choose somewhere you can rest comfortably without distractions. This can be a quiet room, a peaceful outdoor spot or anywhere else that feels calm and soothing.

FOCUS ON YOUR BREATH. Take a few deep breaths, feeling the air moving in and out of your body. Then focus on your breath as it flows naturally, without trying to change it in any way. You can place your hand on your belly to feel the rise and fall with each breath, or pay attention to the sensation of the breath through your nose.

NOTICE YOUR THOUGHTS. As you focus on your breath, you may notice thoughts and feelings rising. This is completely normal! Don't try to push them away or get caught up in them; simply notice them without judgment. Imagine they're clouds passing in the sky or leaves floating down a stream.

RETURN TO YOUR BREATH. Whenever you notice your mind wandering, gently bring your attention back to your breath. You may need to do this many times, and that's okay. Each time you return to your breath, you're practising mindfulness.

PRACTISE REGULARLY. Aim to practise mindfulness for a few minutes each day, gradually increasing the length of your sessions as you feel comfortable. Try incorporating mindfulness into other activities, such as walking or washing dishes, by focusing on the present moment and the sensations in your body.

Remember, mindfulness is not about achieving a certain state of mind or feeling completely relaxed. It's about cultivating awareness and presence in the moment. Give this simple mindfulness plan a try and see how it works for you. With regular practise, mindfulness can help to reduce your stress and anxiety, improve your focus and concentration and promote your overall well-being. Most importantly, it can give you more available energy – something you really need when you're struggling with Long Covid.

5. Breathing

Breathing exercises are beneficial for people with Long Covid because they calm the nervous system, reduce anxiety and stress and improve respiratory function. They can help retrain breathing patterns and increase your lung capacity, alleviating symptoms and promoting overall well-being.

Some popular breathing techniques for Long Covid patients include diaphragmatic breathing, paced breathing and alternate nostril breathing. These techniques stimulate the parasympathetic nervous system via the vagus nerve, lower cortisol levels and improve heart rate variability.

Incorporate these breathing exercises into your daily routine to enhance your well-being and promote relaxation. You can practise these techniques as part of a daily mindfulness practice, or whenever you need to take a few moments to relax and centre yourself.

Within the realms of mental rest,
the seeds of rejuvenation find their
fertile ground. Embrace the stillness,
for it holds the power to nourish your
weary mind and breathe life into
your tired spirit and replenish it.

✳ SIMPLE CALMING BREATHING EXERCISE ✳

✦ Find a quiet, comfortable place to sit or lie down.

✦ Close your eyes and take deep breaths, inhaling through
the nose and exhaling through the mouth.

✦ Place one hand on your belly and the other on your chest.

✦ Breathe in slowly through your nose, feeling your belly expand.

✦ Hold your breath briefly, then exhale slowly through your mouth,
focusing on the belly contracting.

✦ Repeat this deep calming breathing for several minutes to
promote relaxation.

✳ THREE-PART BREATHING ✳

✦ Find a quiet, comfortable place to sit or lie down.

✦ Place one hand on your belly and the other on your chest.

✦ Inhale deeply through your nose, filling your belly, ribs
and upper chest with air.

✦ Exhale slowly through your mouth, releasing tension and stress.

✦ Practise this three-part breathing for several minutes to calm the
mind and body.

✳ NADI SHODHANA: ALTERNATE NOSTRIL BREATHING ✳

✦ Sit comfortably with a straight spine and closed eyes.

✦ Using the thumb of your right hand, block your right nostril.

✦ Inhale deeply through your left nostril and hold your breath.

✦ Using your ring finger of your right hand, block your left nostril and exhale
through the right nostril.

✦ Keeping the left nostril closed, inhale through the right nostril and hold.

✦ Close the right nostril with your thumb and exhale through the left nostril.

✦ Repeat this cycle for several minutes to balance energy flow and reduce stress.

Deep rest – avoiding overload

The importance of deep rest in the realm of Long Covid cannot be overstated. It is a vital sanctuary, a respite for your weary body and mind to find solace and renewal. Just as a tired traveller seeks refuge in a cosy inn along the winding road, you too must seek the haven of rest to restore your vitality.

When resting deeply, time slows its relentless pace and you have permission to surrender to the embrace of tranquillity. Let go of the burdens that weigh upon your shoulders and allow the stillness to cradle you. Within this sacred space, your body rejuvenates, your mind finds clarity and your spirit rekindles its inner flame.

Deep rest is a state of profound relaxation in which your body and mind fully let go of tension, stress, fatigue and other forms of exertion. This state of restful awareness allows your body and mind to enter a deep state of healing and regeneration. It involves slowing down your pace of life, letting go of worries and concerns and taking time to recharge and renew.

During deep rest, the nervous system shifts from a state of sympathetic activation (fight or flight) to parasympathetic activation (rest and digest), so your body can restore and replenish itself. You should find a range of physical and mental benefits, including reduced stress and anxiety, improved sleep quality, increased energy and vitality and enhanced immune function.

STRATEGIES FOR PROMOTING DEEP REST	
Get enough sleep.	You need sufficient sleep for physical and mental health. Aim to get at least seven to eight hours of sleep per night.
Take breaks throughout the day.	Taking short breaks throughout the day can help to refresh your mind and increase productivity. Step away from work or other tasks and engage in a relaxing activity, such as meditation or deep breathing.
Practise relaxation techniques.	Techniques such as meditation, deep breathing and progressive muscle relaxation help to calm the mind and body, reduce stress and anxiety and promote feelings of relaxation and well-being.

Engage in enjoyable activities.	Doing things you enjoy, such as hobbies, reading or spending time in nature, can help to promote relaxation and rejuvenation.
Practise self-care.	Self-care involves taking care of your physical, mental and emotional needs, such as taking a warm bath, getting a massage or practising mindfulness.

Different types of rest are beneficial for several reasons. Let's look at physical, mental and social rest.

Physical rest

Physical rest includes sleeping, napping and moving the body gently, such as getting a massage, stretching and yin yoga. When you're feeling physically tired, physical rest is excellent. Several types of physical rest can be beneficial for promoting relaxation, reducing stress and improving overall health and well-being.

PASSIVE REST involves simply lying down or sitting in a comfortable position then relaxing the body. This can help to reduce physical tension and promote relaxation.

ACTIVE REST involves engaging in low-intensity physical activities, such as gentle stretching, walking or yoga. These activities can help to promote circulation, reduce muscle tension and improve overall physical and mental well-being.

SLEEP is a critical type of physical rest that your body needs to repair and regenerate itself. Getting enough restful sleep can help to improve your cognitive function, reduce stress and support your overall health and well-being. Deep sleep promotes cellular clean-up in the body, which reduces inflammation. A lack of sleep can activate inflammation-related genes, which can considerably burden the immune system.[53] Not getting enough sleep also heightens your cortisol levels. (Hello, stress!)

NAPPING during the day can help to reduce the overwhelming fatigue of Long Covid, improve cognitive function and rest the nervous system. Don't feel guilty for taking naps; just take them as you need.

Mental rest

In the relentless mental battle of the long-hauler, the mind becomes a battleground of fog and fatigue. The need for mental rest is our steadfast companion, beckoning us to seek solace and respite. As I embarked on my journey with Long Covid, I quickly realised that my once-sharp focus had become a blurry haze. My path ahead seemed like an intricate maze with no clear exit.

In that moment of surrender, when I fully embraced the art of letting go, I discovered the power of mental rest. When I realised that pushing myself only deepened the fog, I released the weight of expectations from myself. I granted myself permission to detach from the demands of the outside world and immerse myself in moments of tranquillity and serenity.

Finding solace, even for just a few precious minutes each day, became my sanctuary. I sought refuge in the pages of a good book, letting my imagination transport me to distant realms. The gentle melodies of music were a balm for my weary soul, soothing the frayed edges of my mind. And oh, the joy of nature's embrace! I'd make slow and deliberate walks to the nearby park, inching my way to a circular swing. There, I'd gaze at the sky, the fresh air invigorating my spirit and cleansing the clutter from my racing thoughts.

The practice of mindfulness became my guiding light. I discovered that by anchoring my attention to my breath, I could steady my wandering mind and tap into a wellspring of positivity. Mindfulness became my secret weapon, unlocking the confidence and resilience I needed to face each moment of the journey, one step at a time.

If you're struggling with mental fatigue and brain fog, I highly recommend finding a guided meditation for nervous system rebalancing. My favourite online meditation is 'Trauma release guided meditation for PTSD and chronic stress', by Mindful Waves Studio. You don't have to think about anything, just find a place to lie down and play the YouTube video, following the prompts.

Mental rest involves taking a break from mental activity – such as thinking, planning and problem-solving – and letting your mind relax and recharge. Along with meditation, mindfulness and nervous system work, try deep breathing to reduce stress and promote relaxation. Progressive

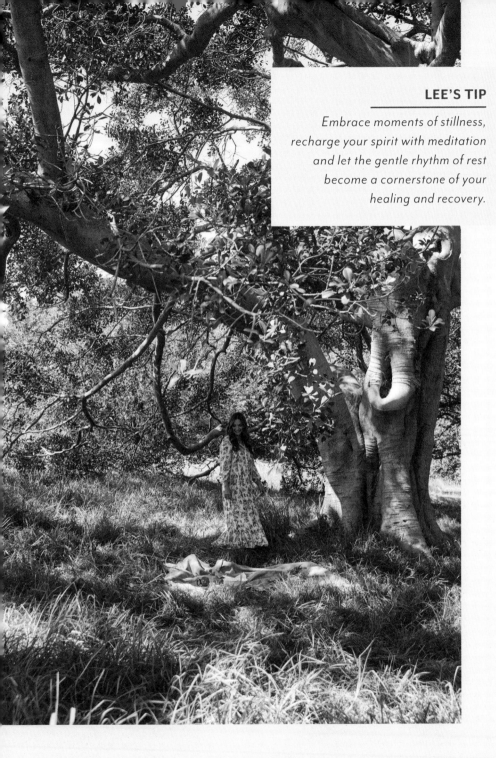

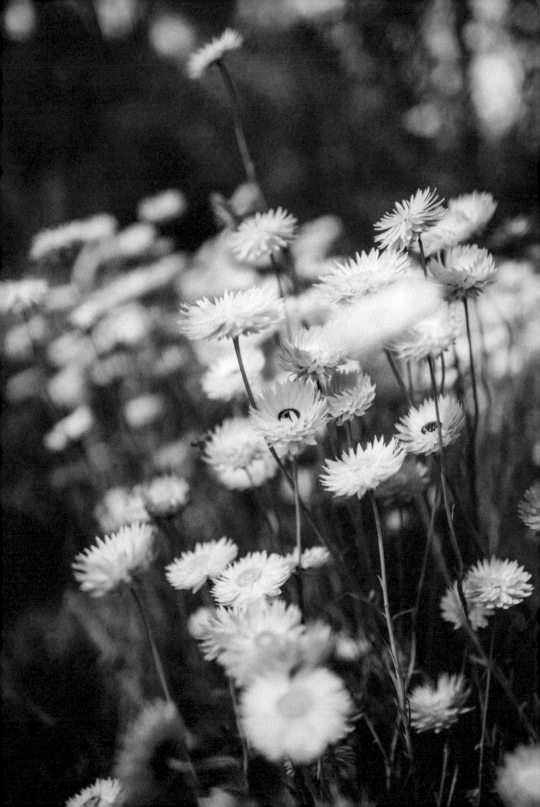

muscle relaxation is another technique that can reduce physical tension and aid relaxation. This involves tensing and relaxing each muscle group in your body, one at a time.

Social rest

Hello, social butterflies and introverted hermits. You're starting to feel better and you want to go out. Well, let's talk about something that might just save you from feeling completely drained after every social interaction – social rest. You know that feeling when you're around certain people and it's like they're sucking the energy out of you? Well, you might need a little break from those energy vampires.

Long Covid has taught me a valuable lesson: not all socialising is created equal. Some people leave you feeling revitalised and ready to conquer the world, while others . . . Well, let's just say they drain your batteries faster than a smartphone with 50 apps running in the background. This is where social rest comes in.

Social rest means giving yourself permission to take a break from social interactions and recharge your social batteries. Be discerning with who you choose to spend your time with and know when it's time to step back and take a breather. Now, I get it – sometimes you can't avoid socialising, like at family gatherings or those obligatory work events where small talk is the main dish. But when it's possible, be choosy about who you surround yourself with.

So how do you practise social rest?

FIND SOME QUALITY ALONE TIME. Embrace the bliss of solitude and engage in activities that make you feel all warm and fuzzy inside. Curl up with a good book, crank your favourite tunes or take a leisurely stroll in nature – whatever floats your introverted boat. And if you're into hobbies that are best enjoyed solo, such as knitting, painting or writing, indulge in them guilt-free.

SET BOUNDARIES. Don't be afraid to communicate your needs and limits to others. It's okay to say 'No' to social invitations or commitments when you need some downtime. Remember, you're not obliged to attend every party or be everyone's social butterfly. Take care of yourself first.

SELF-CARE IS ALWAYS ON THE MENU. Pamper yourself with relaxing activities. Treat yourself to a soothing bubble bath, indulge in a massage or dive into the world of mindfulness and meditation. Find what makes you feel Zen and make it a regular part of your social rest routine.

LIMIT YOUR SOCIAL MEDIA AND TECHNOLOGY USE. I know it sounds crazy, but hear me out. Social media is a never-ending stream of social stimulation and distraction, so take a breather from the constant notifications and scrolling. Unplug for a bit and focus on reconnecting with yourself and the real world.

When you're ready to get back out there, remember the power of social rest. Take breaks, be discerning with your social interactions and give yourself permission to recharge. After all, you deserve to feel energised, not like you've been run over by a stampede of chatty elephants. Here's to finding your social balance and embracing the bliss of solitude! You've earned it, and it will keep you from relapsing into long-hauler fatigue the next day.

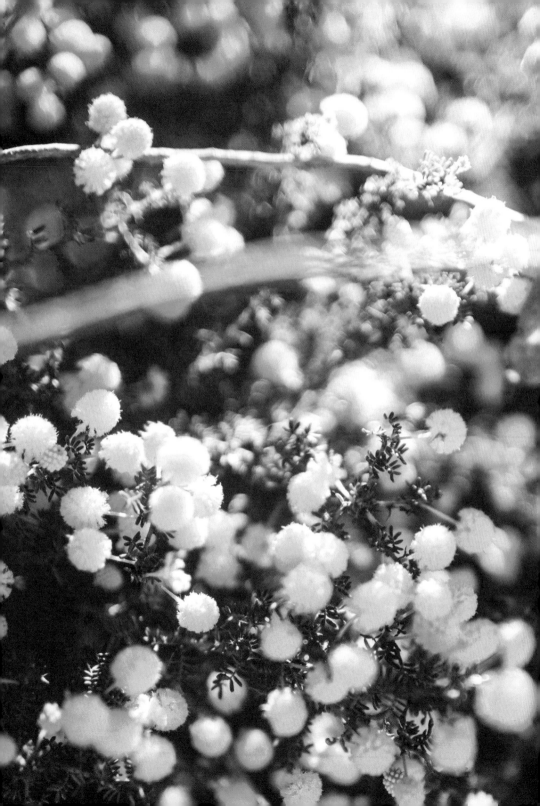

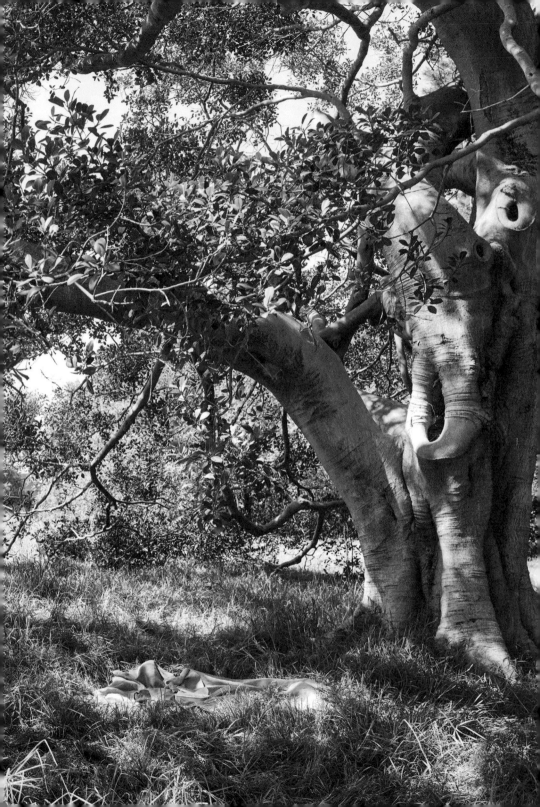

Long Covid may cast its shadows, but your resilience will shine through and lead you to brighter days. You've got this!

Social anxiety, depression and sensory overload

Fellow long-haulers, let's talk about the not-so-fun side of Long Covid: the psychological rollercoaster ride. We all know the physical symptoms can be a real pain, but what about the sneaky social anxiety and depression that tag along for the ride?

Social anxiety is the ultimate fear of being judged or evaluated by others. It's that tiny voice in your head constantly whispering, 'Everyone's watching you, and they're definitely judging you.' You might find yourself avoiding social situations altogether, huddling up in your cosy isolation blanket. It's a lonely place to be, especially when you're already dealing with the physical limitations of Long Covid. But who needs a wild party when you can have a solo Netflix marathon, right?

Social anxiety and depression are common mental health symptoms in people with Long Covid. To help you manage these symptoms, try seeking professional help, practising self-care, connecting with others, practising relaxation techniques, challenging negative thoughts, focusing on the present moment and being patient and kind to yourself. I've been there myself, and I've got some tried-and-tested tricks up my sleeve to tackle those unwelcome feelings.

HELPFUL STRATEGIES FOR SOCIAL ANXIETY	
Try cognitive-behavioural therapy.	This is like having a personal cheerleader in your corner. It helps you identify and challenge negative thoughts and behaviours, replacing them with more positive ones. Think of it as training your brain to be an Olympic gold medallist in positivity.
Get moving.	Who needs a fancy gym membership when you can bust out some dance moves in your living room? Regular exercise, even if it's just a leisurely stroll, can work wonders for your mood because you're giving your brain a natural dose of happy hormones.
Reach out and connect.	Long Covid might make socialising tricky, but that doesn't mean you have to be a hermit. Connect with others who are going through the same journey as you. Virtual support groups and online communities are a great way to combat the loneliness monster.
Relax and unwind.	Deep breathing, meditation and yoga can help calm those racing thoughts and bring some peace to your restless mind. Tap into the world of relaxation and enjoy your own personal spa day, minus the cucumber slices on your eyes.
Sleep like a boss.	Good sleep hygiene is the key to taming depression. Stick to a regular sleep schedule, banish those screens before bedtime and create a cosy sleep sanctuary. You'll be giving your brain a well-deserved vacation.
Feed your mood.	While you can't eat your problems away, a balanced diet can work wonders for your mental well-being. Fill your plate with nutrient-rich, low-histamine foods and wave goodbye to those hangry mood swings.
Seek professional help.	Sometimes, you need a little extra support, and that's okay. Reach out to healthcare professionals or therapists who specialise in treating social anxiety and depression.
Practise self-care.	Treat yourself like the rockstar you are. Take time for self-care activities that bring you joy and relaxation – a bubble bath, a good book or perhaps a guilty-pleasure TV show.

Sleep and nightmares

Long Covid can have a significant impact on sleep. Many people with Long Covid experience disrupted sleep patterns and difficulties falling and staying asleep. I still struggle with sleep and Long Covid nightmares, in which my nightly dreams win the Academy Award for Best Picture every single night. Several factors may contribute to sleep disturbances in Long Covid.

> **PHYSICAL SYMPTOMS ASSOCIATED WITH LONG COVID.** Common symptoms such as fatigue, shortness of breath and muscle pain make it difficult for individuals to get comfortable and fall asleep. Their breathing patterns may also be altered, which can contribute to sleep disturbances. Some people may experience periods of rapid or shallow breathing, which can lead to disruptions in sleep.

> **THE PSYCHOLOGICAL IMPACT OF LONG COVID.** The uncertainty surrounding the illness, as well as its potential long-term effects, can lead to increased stress and anxiety, both of which can negatively affect sleep. The social isolation and feelings of loneliness people experience can also contribute to sleep disturbances.

> **MEDICATIONS USED TO MANAGE LONG COVID.** Medications used to manage pain or inflammation, for example, may cause drowsiness during the day, which then make it difficult to fall asleep at night. After using antihistamines for mast cell issues connected to Long Covid, I found that I needed to take them earlier in the evening so as not to be drowsy the next day. Other medications may have stimulating effects, which is not what you need for sleep.

Unfortunately, sleep disturbances can exacerbate the physical and psychological symptoms of Long Covid. For example, poor sleep can increase your feelings of fatigue and reduce the body's ability to fight infections, which can make it harder to recover from the illness.

Sleep Expert Olivia Rezzolo says, 'Sleep is critical for the production of human growth hormone, the primary catalyst for cellular repair – 70 per cent is produced in slow wave sleep. This means if we are not spending sufficient time in slow wave sleep – ideally 20 per cent of our total sleep time – we compromise our capacity to recover. In a similar light, lack of sleep reduces the activity of natural killer cells – immune agents to hunt and kill invading pathogens – by 28 per cent after just one night.[54] With these agents critical for recovery and prevention of re-infection, it stresses the importance of getting quality sleep – especially when we are recovering.'

Vivid nightmares and disturbing dreams often cause intense fear, anxiety and distress. They usually occur during the rapid eye movement (REM) phase of sleep and can wake you up, leaving you feeling anxious and frightened. Nightmares may be caused by factors including stress, anxiety, trauma, medications (e.g. steroids), sleep disorders and certain medical conditions.

In the case of Long Covid, nightmares can result from the physical and emotional stress your body is under due to your ongoing illness. The anxiety and uncertainty surrounding the illness can also contribute to nightmares.

Not everyone with Long Covid will experience nightmares, but if you do, it can be a distressing symptom that affects your overall quality of life. Seek medical attention and address any underlying medical conditions or medications that may be contributing to your nightmares. Practising good sleep hygiene and relaxation techniques may also help to reduce the frequency and intensity of nightmares.

Reasons for nightmares include the following:

1. Long Covid patients may experience anxiety and depression. These common psychological issues can contribute to nightmares. Anxiety and depression can cause a person's mind to become more active and alert, leading to increased dream activity during sleep. This can lead to nightmares, causing the person to wake up feeling distressed and anxious.

2. Long Covid can disrupt sleep patterns. Symptoms such as coughing, shortness of breath and fatigue can make it difficult to fall asleep and stay asleep. If you're not getting enough restful sleep, your brain is more likely to experience intense and vivid dreams, including nightmares. Olivia says, 'Lack of sleep can increase cortisol, a stress hormone, by 37 per cent after one night of insufficient sleep. This can suppress immune activity and increase feelings of stress, anxiety and fatigue alike.'

3. Long Covid patients may be experiencing PTSD. This is a condition that can occur after a person experiences or witnesses a traumatic event. People with PTSD often have intense and vivid nightmares related to the traumatic event they experienced.

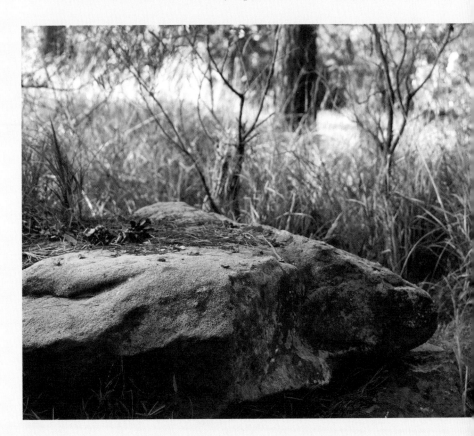

To address nightmares, you need to treat the underlying causes. This can involve treating anxiety and depression through therapy, medication or both. Establishing healthy sleep patterns through good sleep hygiene practices, such as creating a relaxing sleep environment and maintaining a consistent sleep schedule, can also help to reduce nightmares.

If you're experiencing PTSD-related nightmares, therapy and medication can be effective treatments. Cognitive-behavioural therapy, for instance, involves working with a therapist to identify and challenge the negative thought patterns and behaviours that contribute to nightmares. Olivia says, 'Seeking support from a trained professional – therapist – is non-negotiable. Nightmares are a sign of subconscious distress – so even if you feel like you are managing things OK, this is an underlying sign that you need additional support.'

You can also promote restful sleep and reduce the likelihood of nightmares by setting the conditions for sleep. Avoid alcohol and caffeine before bed because they can keep you awake. Also try practising relaxation techniques such as meditation or deep breathing, and creating a relaxing bedtime routine. These activities can help promote feelings of calm and relaxation, making it easier to fall asleep. You may also want to avoid watching or reading anything that could be triggering or upsetting before bedtime.

One important strategy is to establish a consistent sleep schedule, which involves going to bed and waking up at the same time each day – even on weekends. By regulating your body's internal clock, its sleep–wake cycle, you can improve the quality of your sleep. You need to get enough rest to manage Long Covid fatigue. Aim for at least seven to eight hours of sleep each night.

Olivia believes that stress-reducing supplements – adaptogens such as reishi mushrooms and ashwagandha – are helpful too, serving to reduce your anxiety, subsequent nightmares and sleep all in one. Because they mediate the stress response, adaptogens help us feel more relaxed, both night and day. For example, ashwagandha can reduce insomnia and anxiety by 70 per cent.[55]

If your room isn't conducive to sleep, make some changes to your sleeping environment. Try adjusting the temperature or humidity in the room, using blackout curtains to reduce light exposure, or investing in a comfortable mattress and pillows. Avoid stimulating activities, such as using smartphones, tablets and computers, for at least an hour before bedtime. These devices emit blue light that can disrupt sleep and make it harder to fall asleep.

Sleep deprivation and disrupted sleep patterns are associated with increased inflammation in the body. Mast cells, which are involved in the inflammatory response, can contribute to allergic reactions and hypersensitivity. Being sleep deprived may trigger mast cell activation and release inflammatory mediators, which worsens Long Covid symptoms. By prioritising quality sleep, you help to regulate mast cell activity and prevent excessive inflammation.

TIPS FOR QUALITY SLEEP	
Establish a routine.	Stick to a consistent sleep schedule – going to bed and waking up at the same time each day, even on weekends.
Create a restful environment.	Make your sleep environment conducive to relaxation. Have a comfortable mattress and pillow; minimise noise and light disruptions; and maintain a cool, dark and quiet bedroom.
Practise relaxation techniques.	Engage in relaxation before bedtime, such as meditation, deep breathing exercises or gentle stretching. These activities can help to calm your mind and prepare your body for sleep.
Limit stimulants and electronic devices.	Avoid consuming caffeine or stimulating substances close to bedtime because they can interfere with sleep. Minimise your exposure to electronic devices – the blue light emitted by screens can disrupt your natural sleep-wake cycle.
Create a bedtime routine.	Establish a pre-sleep routine that signals to your body it's time to wind down. This can include activities like reading a book, taking a warm bath or practising relaxation.
Ensure a comfortable sleep environment.	Maintain a cool and well-ventilated bedroom, use comfortable bedding and consider using earplugs or an eye mask if necessary.

Remember, everybody's sleep requirements are different, but aiming for seven to nine hours of uninterrupted sleep per night is recommended for optimal health and immune function. By prioritising quality sleep, you're taking a proactive step in supporting your body's natural defence mechanisms, potentially reducing viral load and regulating mast cell activity.

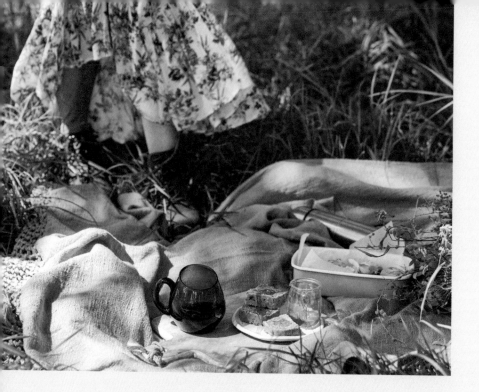

Sensory overload: how to down tools, go back to basics and time out

Let's dive into the wild world of sensory overload. Picture this: you're surrounded by an onslaught of sensory stimulation that's like a rollercoaster ride for your brain. Lights are flashing, sounds are blaring, textures are assaulting your skin and smells are bombarding your nose. It's a chaotic carnival in your head, and you're desperately trying to keep up.

Sensory overload is a sneaky little condition in which you're exposed to more sensory input than your poor brain can handle. It's like your senses are on steroids and they're partying harder than you ever could. This overload can happen in any of your fabulous five senses: sight, hearing, touch, taste and smell.

When you find yourself in the clutches of sensory overload, it's no picnic. You might experience irritability, anxiety, fatigue, headaches, difficulty concentrating or a heightened sensitivity to everything around you. Your senses are throwing a temper tantrum and you're taken along for the wild and chaotic ride, feeling dizzy and disoriented.

Sensory overload is common in Long Covid. If it's a part of your wheelhouse, here are some ways to tame the sensory beast and find your calm amidst the storm.

NIFTY STRATEGIES TO HELP YOU REGAIN CONTROL	
Reduce sensory input.	Give your senses a breather by minimising your exposure to intense stimuli. Lower the volume on those blaring speakers, dim the lights or pop in some earplugs to create a little bubble of peace.
Take a break.	When the sensory madness becomes too much, take a timeout. Find a cosy spot, sit yourself down and take some deep breaths. Focus on the sensation of your breath as it enters and leaves your body – your personal Zen moment in the midst of the chaos.
Unleash your relaxation techniques.	Dive into the world of relaxation and find what works for you. Whether it's deep breathing exercises, progressive muscle relaxation or guided imagery, these techniques can help soothe your stressed-out senses.
Embrace the weighted blanket.	Wrap yourself in the comforting embrace of a weighted blanket. Its warm hug calms your nerves and helps to melt away the anxiety.
Give sensory integration therapy a whirl.	This fancy therapy involves gradually introducing sensory stimuli in a controlled environment, helping your brain get accustomed and build up tolerance to the sensory onslaught. It's like training your senses to be the ultimate superheroes of adaptation.
Seek professional help.	If sensory overload is wreaking havoc on your daily life, reach out to a healthcare provider or therapist. They can offer additional support and suggest specific treatment options that cater to your sensory needs.

Sensory overload doesn't have to leave you feeling like a raggedy old sock. You have the power and discernment to take control, find your restful moments and give your senses the respite they deserve. Life is too short to be constantly bombarded by sensory chaos. Two keys to shortening Long Covid are to calm your senses and reclaim your inner peace.

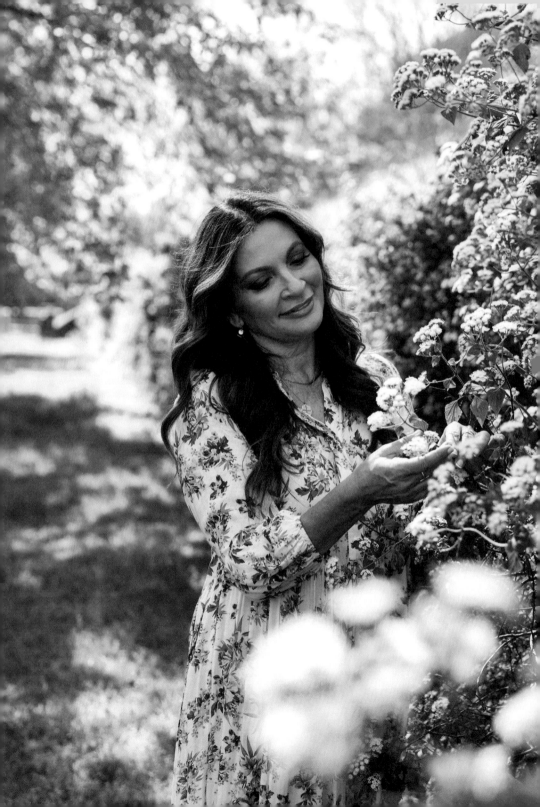

Physical activity supports your long-term recovery, improves your overall health and reduces your risk of long-term complications.

The road to recovery: returning to physical activity

Are you ready to dip your toes into the world of exercise after a bout of Long Covid? Fantastic! But hold your metaphorical horses: we need to approach this with caution. If you're experiencing severe fatigue, particularly post-exertion malaise, don't jump into exercise or push yourself because this can make it worse. Move your body slowly and gently. As you begin to have less tiredness, gradually increase your movement.

Returning to physical activity after experiencing Long Covid is a gradual and often challenging process. The symptoms of fatigue, shortness of breath, muscle weakness and joint pain, which you may experience, can make it difficult to resume your pre-Covid exercise routine. However, incorporating physical activity into daily life is crucial for long-term recovery, overall health improvement and lower risk of long-term complications.

To return to physical activity safely, consider these strategies:

1. Seek out an exercise physiology, physiotherapy or rehabilitation professional. They'll provide personalised guidance based on your specific symptoms and medical history, so you start at a level of physical activity that is safe and appropriate.

2. Start slowly and gradually increase the intensity. Begin with low-intensity activities such as walking, stretching or light resistance training. Listen to your body and increase the amount and duration of the activity based on how you feel. If you like walking, lace up your sneakers and head to the beach or bush. Channel your inner nature enthusiast and indulge in exercise that will bring harmony to your body and nervous system. But here's the twist: if you notice any symptoms making a comeback, pump the brakes. Dial things back and listen to what your body is communicating with you. Don't push through, just try to pace yourself and adjust accordingly until you find your sweet spot.

3. Monitor your symptoms during and after physical activity. If you notice symptoms such as fatigue, shortness of breath or muscle weakness worsen during or after exercise, you need to decrease the intensity or duration of that activity. It's also important to set realistic goals. Start with small, achievable goals and gradually work up to greater challenges.

4. Rest days are crucial for recovery after physical activity. Incorporate rest days into your exercise routine and pay attention to your body's signals when it needs to rest. Focus on low-impact activities such as walking, cycling, swimming or yoga, because high-impact activities may be too intense initially. Also incorporate strength training into your routine to help rebuild muscle strength and endurance. Begin with light resistance exercises, gradually increasing the weight and strength as you progress.

5. Prioritise warming up and cooling down. This helps to prevent injury and reduce muscle soreness. A proper warm-up should include light

aerobic exercise and stretching, while a cool-down should focus on stretching and relaxation. Remember to drink plenty of water before, during and after exercise to avoid dehydration.

6. Listen to your body. Returning to physical activity after Long Covid is a gradual, nonlinear process. If you feel fatigued or weak, you may need to decrease the intensity or duration of the activity and build up again.

7. Give yourself permission to take well-deserved breaks. Always prioritise rest and recovery to avoid setbacks and injuries. Here's a little secret: a relaxing bath with Epsom salts and a splash of lavender essential oil can work wonders for those muscle aches and promote restful sleep. Picture yourself soaking in a fragrant oasis, bidding farewell to any post-exercise discomfort.

With patience, persistence and mindful attention to your body's needs, you can safely reintroduce physical activity into your life. You'll be supporting your long-term recovery, improving your overall health and reducing your risk of long-term complications.

Practising gratitude

In the context of Long Covid, and speaking from personal experience, gratitude is a potent ally in our mental and emotional well-being. Gratitude is like donning a superhero costume and saying a sincere 'Thank you' to all the good things in our lives. It certainly helped me out of my Long Covid depression and social anxiety.

Finding delight in the little things helps when you're being pushed in confronting directions. A warm cup of English breakfast tea feels like a comforting embrace, and a sunny day is like mother nature personally inviting you outside. Suddenly, you're noticing the little miracles that previously went unseen, like a ray of joy shining its light on the ordinary and the everyday.

At its foundation, gratitude is all about appreciating the blessings and magic woven into our lives. But how do we put this transforming art into practice? The choices are as varied as a box of chocolates. We might start a daily gratitude journal by listing three things for which we are grateful. Let the ink on those pages gleam with gratitude, whether it's for the delicious flavour of popping a perfectly ripe blueberry or the laughter shared with a close friend.

Another way to spread the enchantment is to show others your thanks. Thank the good people who have supported or added warmth and love to your life. Let them know how much their presence means to you, whether it's through a sincere conversation, handwritten message or unexpected phone call.

Here's a little known fact: thankfulness can weave its magic even in the most challenging circumstances. Look for the life lessons, the personal development or even the little rays of optimism that poke out of the shadows. Not everything needs to be a lesson; you can rewrite your story from a different perspective.

✳ A MOMENT OF GRATITUDE ✳

I'd like you to spend a moment being totally present. Take in the sights, sounds, smells and sensations dancing around you. You'll find a spring of thankfulness bubbling up when you pay attention to the beauty of the current moment.

Close your eyes, take a deep breath and allow yourself to be filled with appreciation. Embrace appreciation with each inhalation and let go of any pent-up negativity with each exhalation. You can picture the person, location or object you feel most grateful for, and watch as its fascinating energy permeates your being.

Why not spend your entire day in the warm embrace of appreciation? With thankfulness as your compass, spend your day being in the moment, reflecting on what has brought you joy, what went well or what special blessings you have discovered.

Remember, gratitude is a lifelong dance. You may perform flawlessly on some days but stumble on others. Continually put your practice into action and focus on the good, and thankfulness will soon become second nature. Once I started to live with gratitude I noticed life's secret sparkle, as if someone had sprinkled glitter on my everyday experiences. These gratitude goggles revealed hidden blessings and wonders that had always been there, patiently waiting for me to notice them.

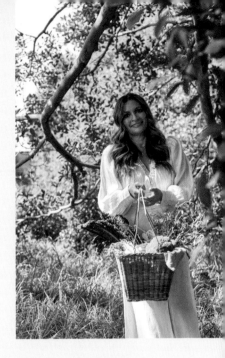

The world transformed before my very eyes. The ordinary became extraordinary and the mundane held a touch of magic. A simple walk in the park became a symphony of colours, scents and sounds. Even everyday encounters with people became a dance of gratitude, as I recognised each person's unique qualities and the contributions they brought into my life.

It wasn't just the external world either. Gratitude reshaped my inner landscape as well. Like a gentle breeze, it swept away the clouds of negativity and replaced them with a sunlit sky of positivity. It was easier to let go of worries and anxieties as I focused on the abundance of goodness that surrounded me.

Practising gratitude became a daily ritual, a joyful treasure hunt. I revelled in the small victories, unexpected joys and quiet moments of peace. My gratitude journal overflowed with scribbles of appreciation, like a love letter to life itself.

The effects extended beyond my own well-being. Gratitude has a contagious nature, spreading its joy like a wildfire. As I expressed my gratitude to others, their faces would light up and their eyes sparkled. Our connections deepened and a sense of warmth and camaraderie enveloped us. Gratitude has a magical power to weave invisible threads of love and appreciation, binding us all in a beautiful tapestry of human connection.

Keeping a sense of humour

Living with an ongoing illness such as Long Covid can feel like navigating a rollercoaster ride with its unexpected twists and turns. Amidst the challenges, a secret weapon can help us conquer the ups and downs: a sense of humour.

HOW HUMOUR CAN HELP IN THE FACE OF LONG COVID	
Humour offers a fresh lens.	Like on a pair of funky glasses, humour reframes our perspective. Suddenly, we see our situation in a new light, finding absurdity in the most unexpected places. We're reminded that there's more to life than our illness, so we can focus on what truly matters.
Laughter tackles stress.	When life throws us lemons, laughter chucks them right back. It has the power to dissolve stress and tension, even in the face of adversity. Laughing is a momentary escape, a breath of fresh air that lightens the burden and helps us carry on.
Make over your mood with giggles.	Humour has a magical effect on our mood. It's our mischievous friend who sneaks in and makes us smile on the toughest days. It injects a dose of positivity, turning frowns into laughter lines and lifting our spirits when they need it most.
It's the immune system's sidekick.	Believe it or not, laughter flexes our immune system's muscles. When battling Long Covid, we need a robust defence against infections and a good laugh can give the immune system an energetic boost.
Comedy connects our hearts.	Laughter builds bridges, connecting us with others on a deep and meaningful level. In the midst of isolation and loneliness, humour is a powerful social glue. It sparks connections, fosters understanding and reminds us that we're not alone on this wild journey.
Reinforce your resilience.	When life knocks us down, humour helps us bounce back. It's our resilient armour, shielding us from despair and empowering us to keep going. With a good sense of humour, we become unstoppable, ready to face whatever comes our way.
Distract yourself from the struggle.	Humour gives us a much-needed intermission from the constant battle with Long Covid. This temporary escape diverts our attention from the challenges and invites us to revel in the joy of the present moment. It reminds us there's still plenty of laughter left to be had.

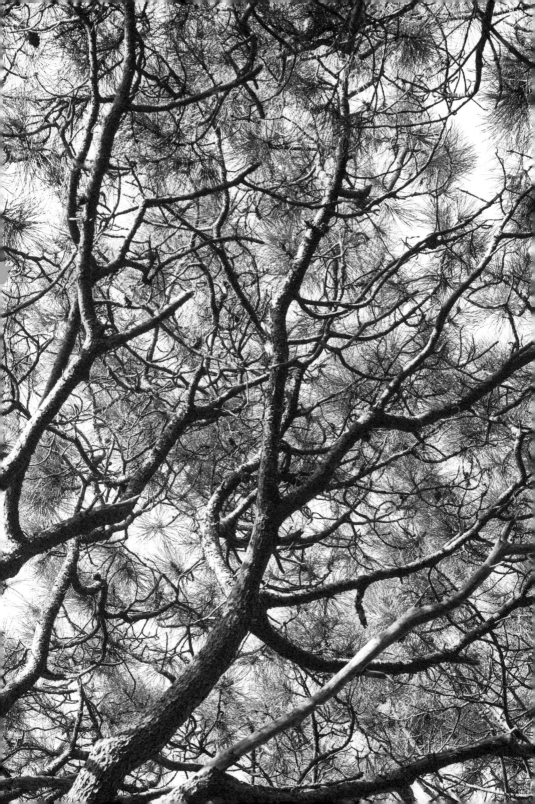

While humour may not have the power to vanquish Long Covid's storm completely, it's a trusty ally that can ease the moments. It won't erase Long Covid, but it will soften its impact, offering us moments of relief and a brighter outlook.

Relapsing and how to quicken recovery times

While everything we've discussed can help you manage Long Covid, you might be wondering what's next and how to avoid experiencing it again. In tackling this topic, as a clinical nutritionist and someone with lived experience, I recommend adopting a holistic approach to your health.

A crucial aspect is managing stress, because stress can weaken the immune system. Everyone has their own way of dealing with stress, but I'd suggest revisiting the various types of rest we discussed earlier (see pages 102–8) and incorporating meditation and pacing into your routine.

It's important to be gentle with yourself throughout the recovery process. Whether it's adjusting your social plans or recognising the need for more sleep, it's okay to prioritise your well-being. Learn to say 'No' and show yourself kindness. You're doing great.

Recovering from an illness is a challenging and lengthy journey, both physically and mentally. It's easy to become frustrated with slow progress or setbacks, but it's crucial to be gentle with yourself during this time.

Here are some tips for recovering from setbacks:

LISTEN TO YOUR BODY, respecting its signals and giving yourself the rest you need if you feel like you're relapsing, which can happen because healing is not linear.

PRACTISE SELF-CARE by focusing on sleep, nutrition, hydration and engaging in activities that bring you joy.

SET REALISTIC GOALS, breaking them down into manageable steps and celebrating each accomplishment.

SEEK SUPPORT from loved ones or healthcare professionals to provide encouragement and assistance.

PRACTISE GRATITUDE to shift your focus towards positive aspects of life. Allow yourself to experience and process your emotions, understanding that they're part of the healing journey.

BE PATIENT WITH YOURSELF, knowing that recovery takes time.

By embracing these principles, you can support your recovery journey and provide yourself with the necessary time and space to heal. Healing takes time, so resist the temptation to compare your progress with others or get frustrated along the way. Instead, celebrate every small victory and trust that, with time and support, healing will come knocking at your door.

One vital aspect of the recovery process is acceptance. Acceptance means embracing the reality of your situation without judgment or resistance. Long Covid may require a slow recovery and setbacks might occur, but accepting these challenges will empower you to better manage your symptoms and work towards regaining your health.

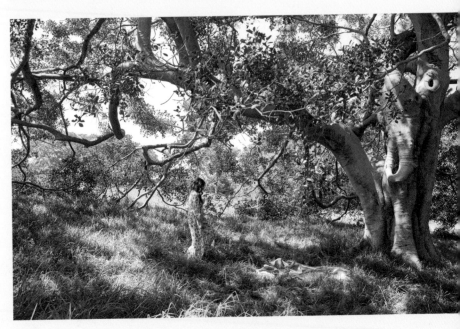

CULTIVATING ACCEPTANCE WITH A TOUCH OF WIT	
Get educated.	Knowledge is power. Learn the ins and outs of Long Covid. By arming yourself with information, you can develop realistic expectations and navigate your recovery journey more confidently.
Embrace mindfulness.	Be here, be now and accept it all. Mindfulness practices like meditation and deep breathing can help you fully embrace the present moment and let go of judgments and worries. Plus, they'll reduce anxiety and stress. So, take a breath and let acceptance be your guide.
Rally your support squad.	Surround yourself with a posse that has your back. Friends, family, support groups and healthcare professionals can offer the encouragement and understanding you need. Sharing your experiences with others who are going through a similar journey can make you feel less alone and provide some much-needed inspiration.
Show yourself some love.	Be kind to yourself, my friend. Treat yourself with compassion and care. Accept that you're doing your best and be gentle when setbacks occur. Remember, you're not perfect, but you're perfectly deserving of love and kindness.
Set goals with a grin.	Keep it real. Set attainable and meaningful goals so you can focus on what truly matters and celebrate each step forward, no matter how small. Progress is progress.
Celebrate like a champion.	Break out the bubbles and celebrate your successes, big and small. Recognise and appreciate the progress you've made on your recovery journey. Let those moments of triumph refuel your sense of acceptance and gratitude.

Remember, acceptance isn't waving a white flag of surrender. It's about acknowledging your situation and taking realistic and compassionate steps towards recovery. So, embrace acceptance with a wink, a smile and the knowledge that you're on the path to healing and are shortening Long Covid. You've got this!

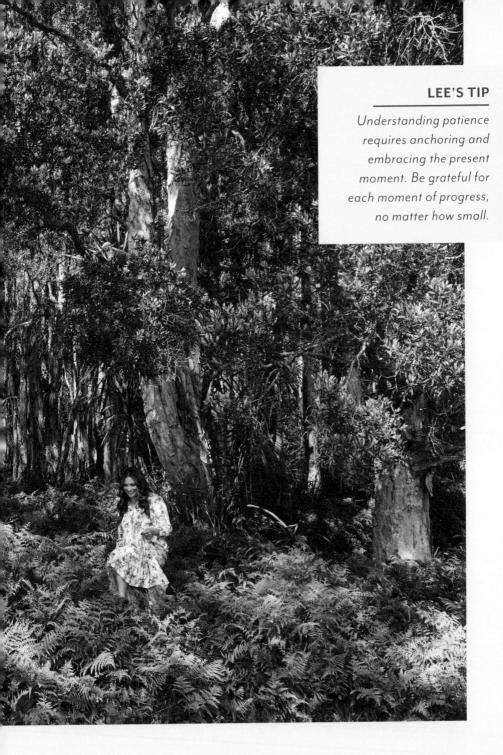

LEE'S TIP

Understanding patience requires anchoring and embracing the present moment. Be grateful for each moment of progress, no matter how small.

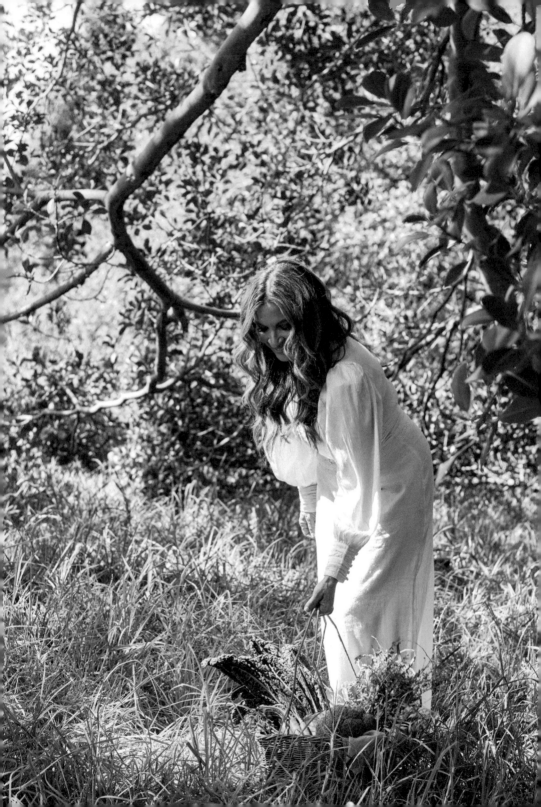

Armed with the right tools, you can navigate Long Covid and its complexities with purpose, one intentional action at a time.

Workbook tools

I've created three valuable resources to support you on your journey of overcoming Long Covid. Let's take a closer look at each one:

1. **MONTHLY SYMPTOM TRACKER.** Keep a close eye on your symptoms with this handy tool. It lets you track and monitor any changes or patterns in symptoms, giving you valuable insights into your progress.

2. **WEEKLY SELF-CARE CHECKLIST.** Prioritise your well-being with this comprehensive checklist. It covers all aspects of self-care, ensuring you're nurturing your mind, body and soul as you navigate your recovery.

3. **PACING DIARY.** Strike the perfect balance between rest and activity using this diary. By planning and tracking your daily routines, you can manage your energy levels effectively and avoid pushing yourself too hard.

With these tools at your disposal, you'll have the support and guidance you need on your Long Covid journey. So, grab your pen and get ready to take charge of your recovery!

Monthly Symptom Tracker

This easy-to-use Monthly Symptom Tracker helps you monitor your progress with Long Covid. It's a valuable tool for understanding your symptoms and communicating effectively with your healthcare team. It can help you identify any changes that may require attention.

MONTH: _____

SYMPTOM	1	2	3	4	5	6	7	8	9	10	11	12
Shortness of breath / difficulty breathing												
Chest pain or tightness												
Muscle or body aches												
Joint pain												
Headache, dizziness												
Brain fog / difficulty concentrating												
Loss of taste or smell												
Insomnia or sleep difficulties												
Heart palpitations / racing heartbeat												
Digestive issues, nausea, diarrhoea												
Skin rashes or lesions												
Hair loss												
Pins and needles												
Low mood, depression												

By performing regular self-evaluations and tracking specific symptoms using the scale from 1 to 5 (with 1 being the lowest and 5 being the highest), you can better understand how Long Covid is affecting you and measure your progress towards recovery. Remember, recovery is a gradual process. Please be patient with yourself as you work towards your goals.

13	14	15	16	17	18	19	20	21	22	23	24	25	26	27	28	29	30	31

MAKING THE MOST OF THE SYMPTOM TRACKER	
Get the tracker.	Have a printed or digital copy of the tracker ready to use. You can download it from my website: superchargedfood.com/longcovid
Set a start date.	Choose a date to begin tracking your symptoms, preferably during a symptom flare-up.
Record your symptoms.	Write the month at the top and document your symptoms daily. Using the provided categories or creating your own, rate the intensity of each symptom on a scale from 1 to 5.
Be specific.	Describe your symptoms in detail. Instead of 'headache', for example, note its type (e.g., dull, throbbing), duration and triggers.
Track changes over time.	Look for patterns or changes in your symptoms to identify triggers or improvements.
Note additional information.	Include medication changes, events or treatments to get a comprehensive view of your well-being.
Review and assess.	Regularly review your tracker to evaluate your progress and share relevant information with your healthcare provider.
Adjust as needed.	Customise the tracker by adding or removing symptoms based on what's helpful for you.
Set specific goals.	Use the tracking data to set recovery goals, such as reducing the severity of symptoms or increasing energy levels.
Develop a progress monitoring plan.	Decide how often you'll evaluate your progress using tools such as symptom tracking apps, daily journals or regular check-ins with your healthcare provider.

Weekly Self-care Checklist

Recovering from Long Covid requires a holistic approach that focuses on your physical, mental and emotional well-being. This Self-Care Checklist is designed to support your healing journey by incorporating daily self-care practices. From nourishing your body to nurturing your mind, this guide empowers you to thrive amidst the challenges of Long Covid.

To get your copy, download the Weekly Self-Care Checklist from my website: superchargedfood.com/longcovid

Long Covid Self-Care Checklist

Week starting: _____
Please check or fill in the appropriate boxes below to
track your self-care activities throughout the week.

PHYSICAL CARE

- O Followed a low histamine diet with plenty of fruits, vegetables, protein and wholegrains
- O Stayed hydrated by drinking at least 1 litre of water per day
- O Engaged in gentle exercises or physical activities
- O Deeply rested and prioritised sleep each night
- O Took supplements or regular medications
- O Practised pacing
- O Practised deep breathing and relaxation exercises
- O Had acupuncture, a massage or other self-care activities

EMOTIONAL WELL-BEING

- O Got into a flow state
- O Practised grounding
- O Practised gratitude
- O Used humour
- O Set aside time for activities that brought joy
- O Did something creative or a hobby
- O Connected with loved ones
- O Sought emotional support from friends, family or support groups
- O Practised mindfulness or meditation techniques to reduce stress and social anxiety
- O Acknowledged and expressed feelings in a healthy way (journalling, therapy)

COGNITIVE STIMULATION

- O Engaged in mentally stimulating activities, reading, puzzles or brain games
- O Limited screen time and took breaks from digital devices to avoid fatigue
- O Practised memory exercises or techniques to support cognitive function
- O Engaged in conversations to stimulate thinking and socialisation

SELF-MONITORING

- O Filled out Monthly Symptom Tracker
- O Used pacing diary
- O Kept a journal to track symptoms, energy levels and any changes
- O Stayed updated with the latest research and information about Long Covid
- O Reflected on progress and any challenges faced during the week
- O Scheduled regular check-ins with my healthcare provider to discuss my symptoms and any necessary adjustments to my care plan

Pacing Diary

Pacing is about listening to your body and adjusting your activities accordingly. Using this diary as a guide, you can identify patterns and make gradual pacing changes to manage your fatigue and symptoms effectively. It's important to prioritise rest and relaxation, and not feel guilty about taking breaks when you need them. Pacing is a gradual process; it may take time to adjust to it. Be patient with yourself.

To get your copy, download the Pacing Diary worksheet from my website: superchargedfood.com/longcovid

TIME	ACTIVITY	ENERGY LEVEL BEFORE	ENERGY LEVEL AFTER	SYMPTOM LEVEL BEFORE
9 am				
10 am				
11 am				
12 pm				
1 pm				
2 pm				
3 pm				
4 pm				
5 pm				
6 pm				

PACING DIARY TIPS	
Date	Record the date for each day.
Time	Note the activity time.
Activity	Record the activity you do.
Energy levels	Rate your energy before and after each activity (on a scale of 1–10).
Symptoms	Note any symptoms during or after each activity (on a scale of 1–10).
Rest breaks	Record rest breaks with their duration and impact.
Reflections	Review your day, with insights and pacing adjustments.

SYMPTOM LEVEL AFTER	REST BREAKS	REFLECTIONS

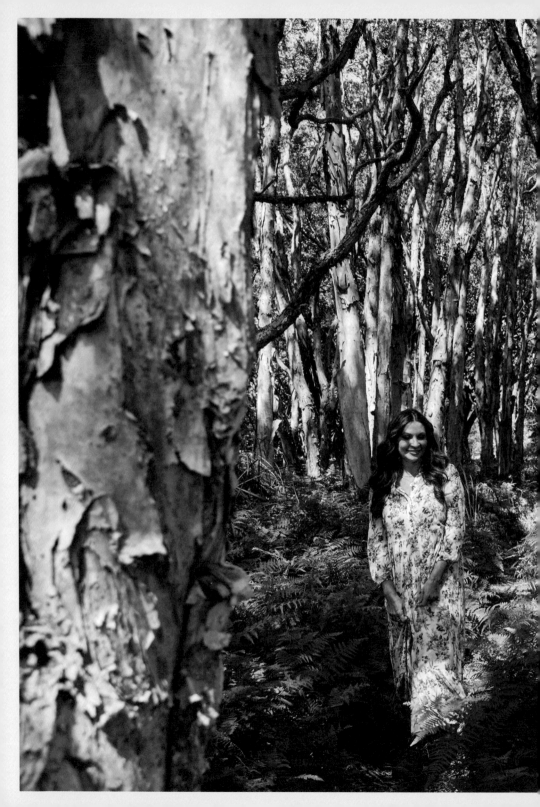

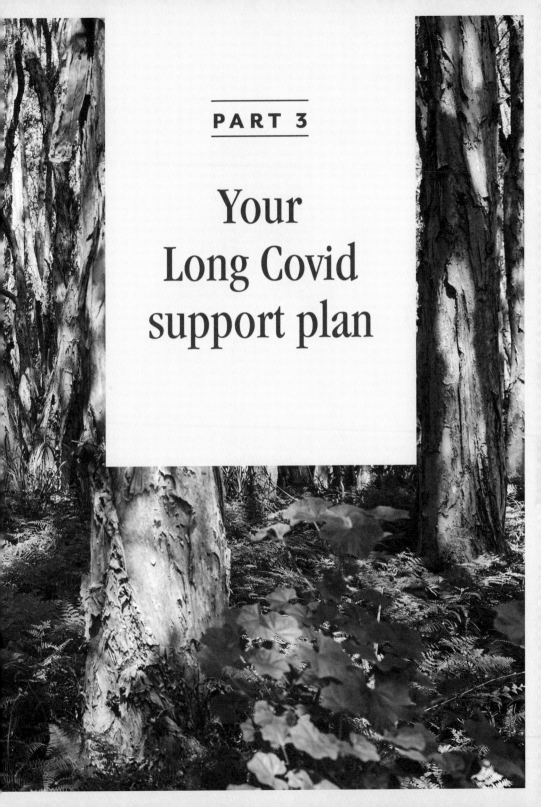

PART 3

Your Long Covid support plan

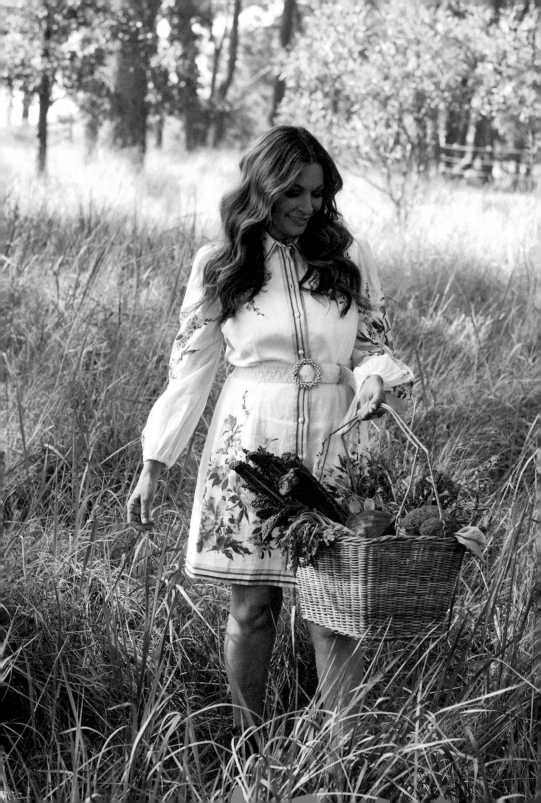

*Natural treatments are
an accelerant to shortening
Long Covid.*

How to heal and shorten Long Covid's lifespan

As we know, Long Covid is characterised by a diverse range of symptoms, which manifest differently in everyone. Symptoms can persist for a long time after the initial acute phase of the COVID-19 infection has subsided. To facilitate the healing process and shorten the duration of Long Covid, you need to focus on these key aspects: managing viral load, addressing inflammation and mast cell activity and alleviating specific symptoms.

Before implementing any symptom management strategies, make sure you undergo the appropriate tests to rule out any underlying conditions that may be contributing to your symptoms. Regular check-ups will help you track your progress and identify any changes in your condition. It's essential to collaborate with a comprehensive healthcare team comprising doctors, physiotherapists, occupational therapists, psychologists and other specialists. They will provide personalised guidance, closely monitor your progress and adapt treatment strategies to your specific needs. Effective communication with your healthcare provider is vital; be sure to inform them of any new or worsening symptoms for their proper evaluation and management. By working together with your healthcare team, you'll optimise your chances of managing Long Covid symptoms effectively.

If you want to support your Long Covid naturally, consider the following factors:

WHY CONSIDER NATURAL SUPPORT FOR LONG COVID?	
Severity and frequency of symptoms	People with Long Covid experience symptoms of varying severity and frequency. Your natural health support should be tailored to address your specific symptoms and their impact on your daily life.
Recovery from organ damage	If you were hospitalised with severe COVID-19 symptoms and are now recovering from organ damage, a holistic approach is helpful. Natural health support can aid in the healing process and promote organ function restoration.
Pre-existing conditions	Long Covid can be particularly challenging if you have pre-existing conditions, such as ongoing respiratory symptoms like shortness of breath and a cough. When accessing natural health support, make sure you consider these conditions and use targeted strategies to alleviate symptoms and enhance your overall well-being. This book contains a general protocol for Long Covid; if you have specific pre-existing conditions, speak to a healthcare provider to ensure these are fully taken into account.
Reactivation of dormant viruses	For some people, Long Covid may lead to the reactivation of dormant viruses. Your natural health support plan should address these viral infections, including Epstein–Barr virus (EBV), chickenpox virus and human herpesvirus 6. You may need specific interventions to manage these viral reactivations effectively.
Hyperinflammation and mast cell activation	Hyperinflammation and mast cell activation can contribute to persistent symptoms such as brain fog, cognitive impairment and fatigue. This protocol focuses on reducing inflammation and regulating mast cell activity through dietary modifications, recipes, targeted supplementation and lifestyle adjustments.
Intestinal microbiota balance	The balance of your intestinal microbiota plays a vital role in your overall health and immune function. Supporting a healthy gut microbiome with immune-based probiotics, prebiotics, my Love Your Gut Synbiotic (which is developed for Long Covid) and a nutrient-rich diet can be beneficial.

Autoimmune disease	If you have an autoimmune disease, you may experience exacerbated symptoms or intermittent flare-ups with Long Covid. Make sure your natural health support addresses immune system dysregulation, inflammation and symptom management specific to your autoimmune condition.
Stress management and nervous system regulation	Long Covid can be emotionally and mentally challenging. Practising stress reduction techniques, relaxation exercises and activities that promote nervous system regulation such as meditation, deep breathing and gentle movement therapies can help to shorten Long Covid's lifespan.
Minimising exposure to toxins	Reduce your exposure to toxins in your environment, such as mould, chemicals and pollutants. Look at creating a cleaner living environment, adopting healthy lifestyle habits and supporting the body's detoxification processes with hydration and an internal cleanser such as my Love Your Gut powder or capsules.
Consideration of current medication regime	When looking at the protocol, consider your current medication regime and speak to your treating healthcare professionals or integrative medicine practitioners to account for any potential interactions or contraindications.
General health optimisation	As well as targeting specific symptoms, this protocol optimises your general health factors. This includes prioritising good-quality sleep, following a balanced and nutritious low-histamine diet, ensuring proper hydration, engaging in regular physical activity suitable for your condition and stage of Long Covid, managing stress and the nervous system, fostering a positive mood and cognition and seeking social support if you need.

Using this protocol as a guide, consult with your personal healthcare professional to work with you on a personalised approach that combines medical guidance, lifestyle modifications, and supportive care to promote your healing and recovery.

While there is no definitive, one-size-fits-all cure for Long Covid, focusing on managing your viral load, regulating mast cell activity, lowering inflammation and providing symptom relief will all contribute to shortening its duration and lessening symptoms over time.

Manage your viral load and regulate mast cell activity

Because Long Covid can be influenced by the persistence of the COVID-19 spike protein in the body,[56] reducing your viral load can contribute to a faster recovery. You can achieve this through antiviral treatments, immune-supporting supplements and natural interventions such as autophagy (see page 153).

Reducing your viral load naturally involves adopting strategies that support your body's immune system and inhibit viral replication. While natural methods may not eliminate the virus completely, they can help in reducing your viral load. Some approaches that may be beneficial are as follows.

Nutrient-rich, anti-inflammatory, low-histamine diet

Consume a well-balanced diet that includes plenty of fruits, vegetables, whole grains, proteins and healthy fats, which are included in the food list (see pages 233–5). Nutrients like vitamins A, C and D plus zinc support the immune function and may help to reduce viral replication. All the recipes in this book are low histamine and will support your recovery from Long Covid (see pages 183–231). Foods that contribute to viral load are sugar – which feeds viruses – and arginine-rich foods such as soy and peanuts. Arginine is an amino acid that is essential in the life cycle of many viruses. Depleting arginine may therefore be an effective therapeutic approach against SARS-CoV-2.[57]

Quercetin is a flavonoid found in fruits and vegetables, such as onions, apples, berries and citrus fruits. It has anti-inflammatory and antioxidant effects that may help to modulate the immune response. Quercetin also blocks the release of histamine from mast cells. Adding quercetin-rich foods to your diet, or considering taking quercetin supplements, can help to stabilise mast cell activity and reduce inflammation. With Long Covid, where mast cell activation and inflammation contribute to symptoms, quercetin is a good option to explore.

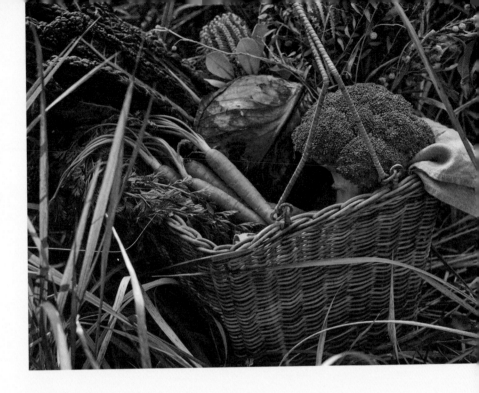

Stay well hydrated by drinking enough water each day. While specific beverages cannot directly reduce viral load, staying properly hydrated is important for your overall health. You'll ensure your body can carry out essential processes efficiently and support the immune system's function. While plain water is the best choice for hydration, some hydrating drinks may provide additional immune-supporting benefits.

Homemade vegetable juices from fresh, low-histamine vegetables such as cucumber, celery, zucchini and lettuce can be hydrating and provide essential nutrients. Make sure you use a blender to make them, so you don't lose all the fibre from the vegetables. Avoid using high-histamine vegetables such as tomatoes, spinach or fermented vegetables.

Healing herbal teas and nourishing drinks

Rooibos tea is a caffeine-free herbal tea made from the *Aspalathus linearis* plant, which has a mild, earthy flavour. This tea is another great source of quercetin and has antihistamine properties.

Herbal teas, such as chamomile, peppermint, ginger and echinacea, provide hydration while also offering potential immune-supporting properties. These teas are rich in antioxidants and may help to support your overall immune health. While chamomile, peppermint, ginger and echinacea are generally considered to be lower in histamine than other herbal options, for people with Long Covid histamine tolerance can vary from person to person. While some individuals with a histamine intolerance or sensitivity may experience symptoms when consuming these herbs, others may tolerate them well.

Herbs and their histamine-related properties

HERBAL TEA	WHERE	BENEFIT
Chamomile tea	Mental health	Calming and soothing effects; typically well-tolerated, calming and soothing; low-histamine
Peppermint tea	Digestion	Relief for digestive issues; low-histamine *Note: Peppermint can exacerbate Long Covid–related acid reflux or GERD in some individuals, so proceed with caution.*
Ginger tea	Digestion, inflammation	Anti-inflammatory, low-histamine; digestive benefits; relief for upset stomach, gastrointestinal issues
Echinacea tea	Immune system support	Generally low-histamine; rare allergic reactions

Remember, listen to your body and observe how you react to these herbs. If you have histamine or mast cell issues, start with small amounts and gradually increase the dosage while monitoring your symptoms. Making a note of these in your Monthly Symptom Tracker can help you identify any triggers or patterns.

DRINK COCONUT WATER. When I was recovering from Long Covid, coconut water was extremely helpful. Coconut water is a natural, electrolyte-rich drink that replenishes fluids and maintains hydration. It also provides essential minerals such as potassium and magnesium, which support proper cell function. This was the one drink that helped the most, especially if I'd been in the heat, which was debilitating at the height of my Long Covid.

HERBAL INFUSIONS CAN HELP. Infusing water with herbs and fruits, such as mint leaves, cucumber, basil or blueberries, adds flavour and may encourage you to drink more water. These infusions are both hydrating and refreshing. Remember, maintaining proper hydration doesn't just depend on beverages, but also on consuming water-rich foods like fruits and vegetables. Be mindful of your overall fluid intake and adjust it according to your activity level, climate and individual needs. As a general rule, aim to drink 35 ml water per kilogram of body weight.

Support your immune system by getting enough sleep

When you sleep your body undergoes restorative processes, such as releasing immune-regulating molecules and producing immune cells. Sufficient sleep allows your immune system to function optimally, enhancing its ability to combat infections, including viral infections.

Adequate sleep can potentially help to reduce your viral load. Sleep deprivation can impair the immune system's ability to effectively control viral replication.[58] In contrast, getting enough sleep supports the immune response, potentially leading to decreasing viral load and clearing the virus more efficiently.

Natural antiviral agents

When it comes to your Long Covid recovery, you may wish to incorporate natural antiviral agents into your routine. While these agents cannot cure or directly target the specific virus causing Long Covid, they possess properties that can support your immune system and potentially inhibit viral replication.

Nature's best antivirals

ANTIVIRAL AGENT	EFFECT	BENEFIT
Garlic	Broad-spectrum antiviral activity	Stimulates immune responses; potential antiviral effects against respiratory viruses
Ginger	Immune-boosting, antiviral activity	Anti-inflammatory benefits; helps to manage Long Covid–associated inflammation
Honey	Antimicrobial and antiviral properties	May inhibit viral replication
Elderberry	Immune-enhancing, antiviral effects	Flavonoids inhibit viral entry and reduce replication
Essential oils (tea tree, eucalyptus, peppermint)	Antiviral properties	Potential antimicrobial, immune-boosting effects; use with caution and proper dilution

Good hygiene practices help with viral load too. Make sure you wash your hands frequently with soap and water for at least 20 seconds. Avoid close contact with individuals who may be contagious.

Lower inflammation

As we learn more about inflammation and its role in the pathogenesis and ongoing nature of Long Covid, you may be able to shorten the duration of symptoms by targeting and reducing excessive inflammation. Chronic inflammation can hinder your recovery process. Natural anti-inflammatory approaches, including specific dietary modifications, supplements and lifestyle adjustments, can help to regulate the body's inflammatory response.

The most important way to do this is to regulate mast cell activity. Mast cells, as you know, are involved in immune and inflammatory responses, and are implicated in the symptoms of Long Covid. Adopting strategies that kerb mast cell activity, such as certain medications, natural supplements and dietary changes, can help you alleviate symptoms and accelerate your recovery.

ALLEVIATE YOUR SYMPTOMS. Long Covid presents a wide array of symptoms, including fatigue, brain fog, respiratory issues, muscle pain and gastrointestinal issues. Getting to the root cause and addressing these symptoms individually can help you shorten the overall duration of Long Covid. Targeted therapies, rehabilitation programs, cognitive training, pain management techniques and respiratory support can all help to manage symptoms.

AVOID EXPOSURE TO ENVIRONMENTAL TOXINS AND POLLUTANTS. Reduce the toxic load on your body by avoiding or minimising contact with the harmful chemicals found in cleaning products, personal care items, pesticides, air pollutants and other potentially toxic substances in your environment.

MAINTAIN A HEALTHY GUT. Your gut helps to eliminate toxins from the body, which reduces inflammation and alleviates symptoms. Supporting a healthy gut microbiome with a balanced low-histamine diet, which is rich in fibre, probiotics and prebiotics, can aid in excreting toxins and promoting overall digestive health.

MINIMISE YOUR EXPOSURE TO TOXIC SUBSTANCES. Certain chemicals, preservatives and medications – both antibiotic and non-antibiotic – can have adverse effects on your gut microbes. Minimising your exposure to these substances can help to preserve the diversity and balance of your beneficial gut bacteria, which are vital in the detoxification process.

SUPPORTING THE LIVER CAN HELP. Your liver is the primary organ for detoxification in the body. Supporting liver health with a nutritious diet, adequate hydration and avoiding excessive alcohol consumption can optimise its function and enhance your body's ability to eliminate toxins.

EAT CRUCIFEROUS VEGETABLES. Vegetables such as broccoli, cauliflower, brussels sprouts and cabbage contain compounds that support the liver's detoxification pathways. Garlic and onions are aromatic vegetables containing sulphur compounds that aid in detoxifying the liver and reducing inflammation. Turmeric contains curcumin, which has potent anti-inflammatory and antioxidant properties that can protect the liver and support its function. Certain herbs also support liver function. Milk thistle, dandelion root and artichoke leaf extract are commonly used to promote liver health and aid in detoxification.

INCORPORATING NATURAL DETOXIFICATION PRACTICES. Fill your daily routine with practices that help your body eliminate toxins: staying hydrated, consuming antioxidant-rich foods, using Love Your Gut Diatomaceous Earth powder or capsules, engaging in regular exercise, and promoting sweating with saunas (if you're okay with heat) or physical activity.

TAKE ANTI-INFLAMMATORY SUPPLEMENTS. Supplements with anti-inflammatory properties include omega-3 fatty acids, curcumin (found in turmeric), resveratrol (found in grapes and red wine) and ginger. Omega-3 fatty acids are found in fatty fish (such as salmon, mackerel and sardines), flaxseeds (linseeds) and chia seeds and have potent anti-inflammatory effects. They help to regulate the body's immune response and can reduce inflammation in different body tissues.

You can take omega-3 supplements, such as high-strength clean fish oil, to ensure your intake is adequate. Curcumin, a compound found in turmeric, has powerful anti-inflammatory properties. It inhibits inflammatory enzymes and mediators in the body. Consider adding turmeric to your diet or taking curcumin supplements to support your body's natural anti-inflammatory mechanisms. Ginger is a spice with anti-inflammatory properties. It contains bioactive compounds that can help to alleviate inflammation and reduce oxidative stress in the body. Incorporating fresh ginger into meals or consuming ginger supplements may provide some anti-inflammatory effects.

When taking medications, please follow your healthcare professionals' guidance and use them only as prescribed. Managing medication properly can minimise unnecessary exposure to potentially harmful substances and reduce the burden on your body's detoxification pathways.

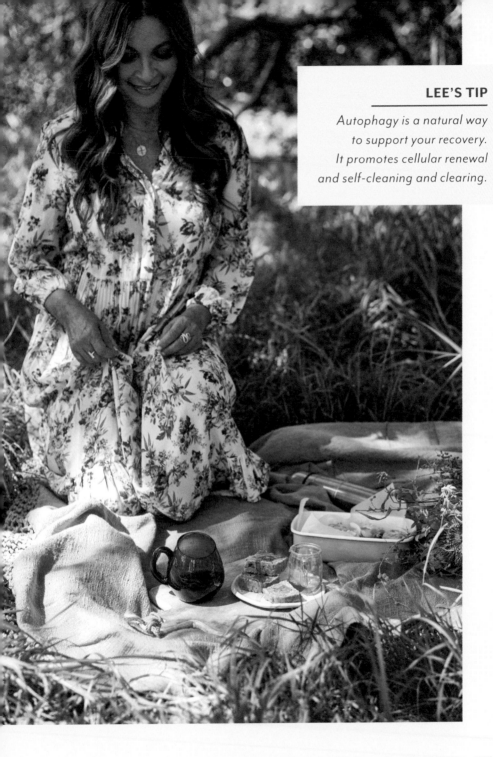

LEE'S TIP

Autophagy is a natural way to support your recovery. It promotes cellular renewal and self-cleaning and clearing.

Autophagy and intermittent fasting

Autophagy is a fundamental cellular process that maintains cellular health and balance. It operates by selectively breaking down and recycling damaged or dysfunctional cellular components, such as proteins, organelles and pathogens. The term 'autophagy' originates from the Greek words *auto* meaning 'self' and *phagein* meaning to 'eat', reflecting the self-consuming nature of the process. With viral infections like Long Covid, autophagy has several benefits, particularly in reducing viral load and influencing the course of the disease.

An important aspect of autophagy is that it can selectively target viral components for breaking down. By eliminating viral proteins and nucleic acids, autophagy helps to decrease the viral load of infected cells, slowing down viral replication. Autophagy also regulates the immune response against viral infections. It helps viral antigens become visible to immune cells like T cells and natural killer cells, thereby boosting the effectiveness of the body's immune response against the virus.

Autophagy also contributes to regulating inflammation, a critical factor in Long Covid. Excessive inflammation, as we know, can lead to tissue damage and prolong the recovery process. By removing damaged cellular components and reducing the release of pro-inflammatory molecules, autophagy helps to mitigate inflammation and promote healing. It also helps to maintain cellular energy balance. In Long Covid, cellular stress and energy depletion are common. Autophagy recycles degraded cellular components and provides nutrients to cells. This supports the function of the cells and enhances their overall health.

Autophagy also clears damaged mitochondria, those energy-producing organelles within cells. By clearing out these damaged organelles, autophagy helps the mitochondria work optimally, which can alleviate fatigue and weakness, both frequently experienced symptoms in Long Covid.

Caloric restriction, particularly through intermittent fasting, is a powerful tool to promote autophagy. Some studies suggest that this dietary pattern could potentially reduce inflammation and improve immune function, both of which are relevant to Long Covid.

Intermittent fasting can offer various health benefits to individuals, including not only weight loss but also improved circadian rhythms, immune cell migration, fewer inflammatory factors and better microbial diversity. Intermittent fasting can exert anti-inflammatory effects while also protecting against oxidative stress. Intermittent fasting can improve your immune function by increasing your body's production of certain immune cells, including natural killer cells and T cells, and decreasing levels of pro-inflammatory cytokines, which are associated with chronic inflammation.

My book and online program *Fast Your Way to Wellness* has detailed information and recipes on intermittent fasting. You can find it on my website: superchargedfood.com

Certain plant compounds, such as resveratrol, quercetin and spermidine, can enhance autophagy. These compounds are found in foods such as red grapes, onions, green tea and wheat germ. Including these foods in your diet can support autophagy in your body; however, green tea can be troublesome for some due to the caffeine component.

You should approach caloric restriction and intermittent fasting with caution, especially if you have underlying health conditions or are taking medications. By restricting feeding to shortened windows, you can effectively stimulate the removal of damaged mitochondria within the body. Fasting promotes the turnover of damaged cells in the body, creating space for new and healthy mitochondria and cells to grow. Embracing fasting as a strategy supports the body's natural mechanisms for regeneration and rejuvenation, improving your vitality and well-being.

✳ REST AND PACE YOURSELF ✳

✦ Allow yourself time for ample rest and prioritise sleep to aid in the recovery process.

✦ Listen to your body and avoid overexertion. Gradually increase your activity levels as tolerated.

✦ Use techniques such as pacing, where you balance activities and rest to manage your energy levels effectively.

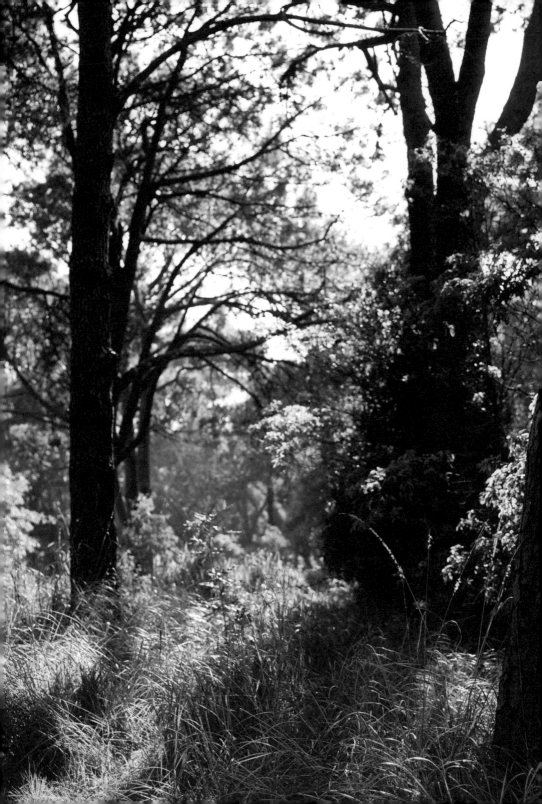

Minimise your viral and toxic loads, and embrace foods that are nutrient dense and gut friendly to support healing.

Managing symptoms

Managing Long Covid symptoms can take a multifaceted approach that focuses on addressing specific symptoms and promoting overall well-being.

Strategies to manage Long Covid symptoms

Everyone's experience with Long Covid is unique and recovery timelines can vary. Patience, persistence and collaboration with healthcare professionals all help in managing your symptoms, promoting healing and potentially shortening Long Covid.

Current scientific research and medication for early intervention and prevention

Using medications should be based on clinical judgment and in accordance with the prescribing guidelines of your healthcare professionals. You'll find a list of medications and research on my website: superchargedfood.com/longcovid

SYMPTOM	STRATEGY
Fatigue and weakness	◆ Pace yourself and prioritise rest breaks throughout the day. ◆ Practise good sleep hygiene and ensure you get enough restorative sleep. ◆ Gradually increase physical activity and exercise under the guidance of a healthcare professional or physiotherapist. ◆ Learn and implement energy-saving strategies in your daily activities. This includes prioritising tasks, delegating responsibilities and using energy-efficient movement patterns. ◆ Communicate your needs and limitations to your family, friends and employers, fostering their understanding and support.
Breathlessness and chest discomfort	◆ Practise deep breathing exercises to improve lung capacity and relaxation (see pages 99–101). Consider pulmonary rehabilitation programs to enhance your lung function. ◆ Avoid triggers that worsen breathlessness, such as allergens or pollutants.
Brain fog and cognitive difficulties	◆ Break tasks into small, manageable chunks to prevent cognitive overload. ◆ Use organisational tools, such as calendars, reminders or apps, to aid your memory and task management. ◆ Play cognitive exercises, such as puzzles or brain games, to promote mental agility.
Joint and muscle pain	◆ Practise gentle stretching exercises and low-impact activities, such as yoga or tai chi, to improve flexibility and reduce pain. ◆ Apply heat or cold packs to alleviate muscle or joint discomfort. ◆ Consider physiotherapy or occupational therapy for targeted pain-management strategies.
Anxiety and depression	◆ Seek emotional support with counselling, therapy or support groups. ◆ Practise stress-management techniques, such as deep breathing, meditation or mindfulness. ◆ Do activities that bring joy and promote your mental well-being, such as hobbies, creative outlets or spending time with loved ones.
Gastrointestinal symptoms	◆ Follow a gut-friendly, low-histamine diet rich in fibre, fruits and vegetables to support gut health. ◆ Stay hydrated and consume enough fluids throughout the day. ◆ Consider working with a clinical nutritionist or dietitian to identify any trigger foods and develop a personalised dietary plan.
Autonomic dysfunction (e.g. dizziness, heart rate fluctuations)	◆ Stay hydrated and ensure adequate salt intake, if recommended by a healthcare professional. ◆ Avoid sudden position changes and be careful when standing up to prevent dizziness or light-headedness. ◆ Engage in activities that promote balance and improve autonomic function, such as vestibular rehabilitation (balance exercises).

Nutritional protocol and support plan

As a qualified clinical nutritionist, I believe you should have a comprehensive nutritional protocol and support plan to manage Long Covid. Proper nutrition supports the immune system, promotes recovery and alleviates symptoms.

My nutritional protocol focuses on providing you with essential nutrients, supporting gut health, reducing inflammation, calming mast cell activation, minimising viral and toxic load and optimising your overall well-being. You can either implement this tailored nutritional plan on its own or with your existing healthcare plan. It will enhance your resilience, improve your energy levels, support your body's healing process and shorten the lifespan of Long Covid.

You'll be incorporating foods that not only make it easier for your gut to digest, but will make you feel lighter and possibly less fatigued. Some of my favourite gut-loving meals are steamed, sautéed, stewed or roasted vegetables; vegetable broths; low-histamine, colourful and fibre-rich fruits and vegetables; and gluten-free grains. Eating foods high in polyphenols helps to improve the gut's mucus layer and regulate the immune system.

Flick through to the recipes and mark your favourites to try (see pages 183–231).

During my recuperation from Long Covid, I worked with Sulin Sze, who is a naturopath and herbalist from Herbalwell.com.au. When it comes to natural remedies, herbs or supplements that can help to alleviate the symptoms of Long Covid, she recommends supplementing with herbs and nutrients to support the physical symptoms of Long Covid. Shifting to an anti-inflammatory diet helps to counteract the qualities of Long Covid, which she says generates dampness and heat internally, driving inflammatory processes that negatively impact the cardiovascular system.

About the links between Long Covid and the gut, Sulin advises, 'I always nourish gut mucous membranes too with herbs like aloe vera.' You can support your cardiovascular health with herbs and supplements such as Japanese knotweed (*Reynoutria japonica*), schisandra (*Schisandra chinensis*) and garlic (*Allium sativum*).

While people's nutrient status varies, some supplements Sulin prescribes for Long Covid symptoms are vitamin C, rutin, quercetin and echinacea – these all improve your innate antiviral response.

She also prescribes magnesium in bisglycinate form, including calcium, vitamin B6 and selenium. To support mitochondrial health and coenzyme Q10 levels, she uses Co-Q10 and sometimes NAC. She says, 'I use a combination of alpha lipoic acid, alpha-tocopherols, liposomal vitamin D3, vitamin C and chromium picolinate if there is strong fatigue, sugar addiction or insulin issues. Turmeric and ginger are also great to relieve inflammation.'

While eating a balanced healthy diet and making lifestyle changes can certainly help, if you're struggling with lingering symptoms, supplements may benefit you. The following is the supplement protocol I have formulated, which has helped so much in my own personal recovery and management of Long Covid.

Because everyone's Long Covid journey is different, before supplementing you should speak to your healthcare practitioner to ensure you're taking the correct things for you. Always follow the dosage instructions on the label and coordinate with your healthcare provider. For further nutritional help, why not join my Long Covid online program? You'll find it at superchargedfood. com/longcovid. I am also available for personalised clinical nutritional consultations: lee@superchargedfood.com

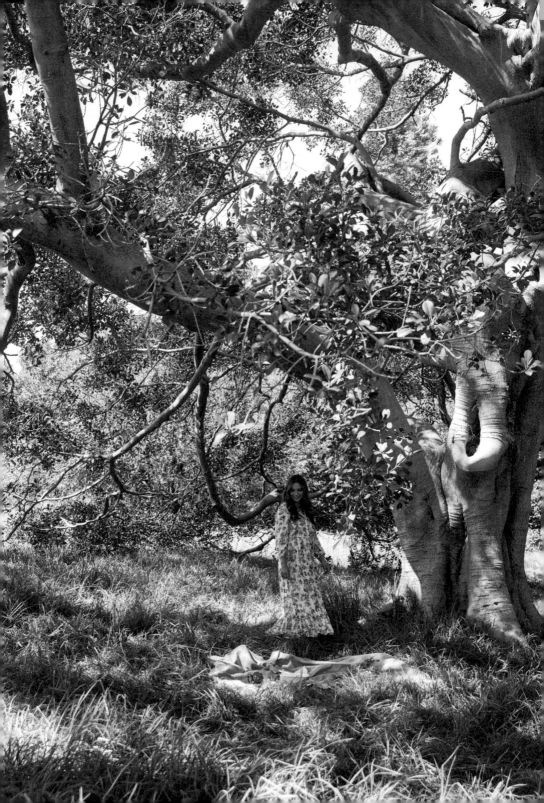

Lee's Long Covid unmasked supplement and nutritional protocol

Love Your Gut products are available from my website: superchargeyourgut.com

WHAT	WHERE	WHY	SOURCE
Vitamin A	Olfactory epithelium health	Protective barrier against infection in the nasal cavity; crucial to our sense of smell and production of mucus	Sweet potatoes, carrots, leafy greens, liver
Vitamin B1 (thiamine)[59]	Supports immune function, energy production	Prevents inflammation, immune system regulation, energy production	Whole grains, legumes, nuts, seeds
Vitamin B6[60]	Deficiency linked to compromised immunity	Supports immune response; enhances the body's defence against viral pathogens	Fish, poultry, fortified cereals
Vitamin B12	Essential for nerve cell health, smell receptors	Deficiency impairs sense of smell and neurological symptoms	Meat, fish, eggs, dairy products
Vitamin C[61]	Antioxidant supporting immune function	Reduces inflammation, boosts antiviral response	Berries, leafy greens, capsicum
Vitamin D[62]	Supports immune function, respiratory health	Deficiency linked to increased infection risk; helps support lung tissues and reduce inflammation; clears persisting viral fragments and reduces autoimmunity; important in brain fog and POTS symptoms	Sun exposure, fatty fish, fortified dairy products
Liposomal vitamin D3	Enhances immune support	Supports immune function; improves outcomes in respiratory infections	Egg yolks, liver, oily fish (tuna, salmon, mackerel, herring)
Antioxidants	Protect cells from oxidative damage	Reduces inflammation in the olfactory system	Vitamin C: berries, leafy greens; vitamin E: nuts, seeds
Bromelain	Natural antihistamine, reduces inflammation	Alleviates respiratory distress and may reduce spike protein in the body	Pineapples

WHAT	WHERE	WHY	SOURCE
Co-Q10[63]	Antioxidant, reduces oxidative stress	Reduces inflammation, supports recovery; may help improve heart function and reduce symptoms of POTS	Kidney, liver, fatty fish, chicken, beef, broccoli, cauliflower
Curcumin	Anti-inflammatory, antioxidant	Promotes digestive wellness and may reduce spike protein in the body	Turmeric*
Diatomaceous earth	Supports gut health, detoxification and energy	Eliminates viruses, bacteria and fungi, and improves digestion; source of fatigue-fighting iron; improves hair, skin and nail health	Love Your Gut Diatomaceous Earth*
Fulvic humic concentrate	Supports gut integrity, microbiota and energy	Beneficial after viral infections, aids leaky gut, energy production	Love Your Gut Fulvic Humic Concentrate*
Glutathione	Powerful antioxidant, immune support	Reduces oxidative stress, anti-inflammatory	Almonds, turmeric, asparagus, milk thistle
Love Your Gut Synbiotic (LC)	Probiotic and prebiotic, digestive enzyme and dietary fibre blend for the gut	Supports healthy gut microbiome, immune function, supports Long Covid	Love Your Gut Synbiotic (LC)
High-strength lyprinol[64]	Anti-inflammatory properties	Supports pericarditis relief	High Strength Lyprinol
Lumbrokinase	Fibrinolytic enzyme, improves blood flow	Enhances fibrinolysis, reduces clotting risk	Lumbrokinase
Magnesium[65]	Cellular function, inflammation regulation	Prevents progression of COVID-19 and Long Covid	Pumpkin seeds, chia seeds, almonds, spinach, cashews, peanuts
Nattokinase	Fibrinolytic enzyme, enhances circulation	Breaks down fibrin, improves blood flow; suppresses viral replication, reduces inflammation	Natto
N-acetylcysteine (NAC)[66]	Precursor to glutathione, immune support	Suppresses viral replication, reduces inflammation	Beef, turkey, eggs, fish, nuts

WHAT	WHERE	WHY	SOURCE
NAD (nicotinamide adenine dinucleotide)	Cellular repair, antioxidant, energy production	Supports mitochondrial function, immune response	Milk, sardines, salmon, tuna
Omega-3 fatty acids	Anti-inflammatory properties	Reduces inflammation, supports immune health	Fatty fish, flaxseeds (linseeds), chia seeds
Polyphenols[67]	Antioxidant, anti-inflammatory properties	Supports endothelial health; reduces oxidative stress	Berries, dark chocolate, olives, apples, grapes, onions, broccoli, turmeric
Quercetin[68]	Antioxidant, anti-inflammatory, spike protein binding	Stabilises mast cells; interacts with spike protein	Dill, onions, apples, capers, berries
Zinc	Essential for immunity, taste, smell	Prevents impaired taste and smell	Oysters, hemp seeds, pumpkin seeds, beans, nuts, animal protein

* Available at superchargeyourgut.com

Formulations

To support my pericarditis, because I couldn't take colchicine, I took Rn Labs Mito-Charge for two months. This formula aids cardiac function and helps to support healthy mitochondrial energy production, sleep, energy, fatigue and muscular recovery after exercise. The magnesium in this formula is a critical factor in producing adenosine triphosphate (ATP), which provides energy to the muscles. I alternated between this and Metagenics Cardio X, which contains magnesium bisglycinate, activated B2, B12, taurine, calcium amino acid chelate, P5P, chromium, activated folate and selenium, until I improved, which took about three months.

To support my MCAS, I currently take Bioceuticals Histammune Clear. It contains quercetin, protease 6, vitamin C, rutin, hesperidin, bromelain and P5P. I also take an oral supplementation of the enzyme diamine oxidase (DAO) before meals to improve my histamine-related symptoms.[69]

Supportive herbal medicines

Herbal medicine is tailored to your individual needs, symptoms and constitution, considering factors like robustness or sensitivity. For immune regulation, medicinal mushrooms such as reishi and shiitake, as well as herbs such as astragalus, garlic, echinacea, elderberry and cat's claw, are commonly used.

If you have adrenal fatigue, burnout and depression, herbal adaptogens such as rhodiola, ashwagandha (withania), liquorice and Siberian ginseng can be beneficial. These herbs help the body adapt to stress, increase energy levels, stabilise mood, improve cognitive function and reduce depression and anxiety.

Herbs such as turmeric, Baikal skullcap, feverfew, ginger, willow bark, frankincense, corydalis and nigella can help to reduce inflammation and alleviate pain.

Certain herbs possess antioxidant properties, which can be beneficial for your overall health. Examples include green tea, maritime pine, rosemary, pomegranate and bilberry. These herbs help protect against oxidative stress and support the body's natural defence mechanisms.

Some herbs support cognitive function: bacopa, schisandra and ginkgo have potential cognitive benefits.

Long Covid has potential effects on various body systems. Herbal medicine aims to address specific actions and support the body's recovery. Adaptogens, nervines, neuroprotective herbs, antidepressants, anxiolytics, adrenal support herbs and nutritive and tonic herbs are often considered.

Popular adaptogens such as ashwagandha, *Rhodiola rosea* and holy basil can increase your energy levels, stabilise mood and reduce stress. Nutritive and tonic herbs replenish essential minerals and vitamins that may have been depleted during your illness. Bitter tonics, such as gentian and dandelion root, can aid in recovery by stimulating your appetite and digestion.

TAKE A HERBAL APPROACH TO PEM. In traditional healing systems, fatigue and lethargy are regarded as natural and protective responses the body initiates to ensure it gets enough rest and recovery. These symptoms reflect the continuing impact of COVID-19 infection on our physiology. Rather than attempting to boost energy or push the body into exertion when it requires rest, Sulin recommends focusing on supporting the adrenals, adrenal hormones, sleep and stress resilience.

PROMOTE SLEEP. Certain herbs such as balm (*Melissa officinalis*), St John's wort (*Hypericum perforatum*) and hops (*Humulus lupulus*) can be beneficial for promoting restful sleep, facilitating the body's restoration and repair processes. You should also minimise physical exertion and avoid unnecessary stress, because these can contribute to feelings of exhaustion and fatigue. By prioritising rest and supporting the body's natural recovery mechanisms, you can help to alleviate these symptoms and aid in the healing process.

TAME INFLAMMATION. Given the inflammation associated with Long Covid, herbs with anti-inflammatory properties can be beneficial. Albizia, arjuna, cat's claw, echinacea, ginger and turmeric are all herbs that may help to reduce inflammation.

ADDRESS POTENTIAL VIRAL INFECTIONS. Herbs with antiviral properties include echinacea, garlic, lemon balm, reishi and turmeric, and liquorice has antimicrobial properties. Sulin advises, 'For Long Covid the virus may have inhibited the recovery response, so you've got an issue with viral persistence in the body. Echinacea (*Echinacea purpurea*) is especially good here as it enhances your ability to inhibit viral infections.' To repair and nourish the lungs, she uses mullein (*Verbascum thapsus*).

PROTECT YOUR MICROVASCULATURE. The presence of antioxidants is important for this. Herbs such as bilberry, green tea, rosemary and turmeric possess antioxidant properties.

SUPPORT YOUR IMMUNE SYSTEM. Herbs such as liquorice (*Glycyrrhiza glabra*), astragalus (*Astragalus membranaceus*) and cang zhu (*Rhizoma atractylodis*) are commonly used for immune support. Herbs should be prescribed with caution, however, because some may potentially amplify the cytokine storm associated with the virus, leading to more severe symptoms.

WHILE THE USE OF ANDROGRAPHIS (*Andrographis paniculata*) has been widely discussed in the naturopathic community, the research is not yet conclusive and there are concerns about its potential side effects.

PROTECT YOUR HEART AND STIMULATE YOUR CIRCULATION. Cardioprotective and circulatory stimulant herbs such as hawthorn, ginkgo, ginger and garlic can help if you have heart or circulatory abnormalities. They may also improve cognition.

BANISH BRAIN FOG. Herbal medicine can help to address brain fog by improving circulation to the brain and aiding in the removal of toxic debris. Naturopaths often use ginkgo (*Ginkgo biloba*) and rosemary (*Salvia rosmarinus*) for their potential cognitive-enhancing properties. Ginkgo supports cerebral blood flow, which can improve oxygen and nutrient delivery to the brain. This can contribute to clearer thinking and improved mental alertness. Rosemary has neuroprotective effects and may help enhance your memory and focus.

As well as herbal remedies, naturopaths also consider dietary factors that may contribute to brain fog. They'll assess your dietary allergies and intolerances and eliminate trigger foods, which can have a positive impact on cognitive function. By identifying and avoiding foods that may cause adverse reactions, naturopaths aim to reduce inflammation and optimise brain health.

During my conversation with Sulin, she highlighted several observations. Initially, in response to the pandemic outbreak, she saw a surge in the use of antiviral herbs such as lemon balm (*Melissa officinalis*), St John's wort (*Hypericum perforatum*), elderberry and liquorice root (*Glycyrrhiza glabra*). Immune-supporting herbs such as echinacea (*Echinacea* spp.), andrographis (*Andrographis paniculata*) and astragalus (*Astragalus membranaceus*), as well as vitamins C and D, were widely utilised to enhance immune function.

While these approaches proved helpful in reducing the severity and duration of the initial infection, they were not sufficient on their own. It was crucial to address the nature of the disease. COVID-19 is characterised by heat and inflammation. Sulin noticed significant variations in individual responses to COVID-19 infection, indicating that the body's response goes beyond the viral pathogen itself. Instead, a sequence of events specific to each individual occurs post-infection. The more heat and damp in someone's internal body, the more severe the symptoms. COVID-19 can destabilise and inflame our internal environments.

When considering herbal medicines, know that they have potential interactions with pharmaceutical drugs; it's important to get professional guidance from qualified herbalists or naturopaths. These practitioners can assess your individual constitution and determine the appropriate herbal remedies that align with your specific needs. The dosage of herbal medicines is critical because it can determine their effectiveness or potential harm, and a healthcare practitioner can make adjustments as necessary.

Understanding the best time to take herbs, whether with food or before/after meals, will maximise their benefits. Seek guidance from a qualified healthcare practitioner when dealing with histamine- and mast cell–related issues. By working closely with a knowledgeable practitioner you can ensure your herbal medicine is tailored to your unique requirements, promoting their safe and effective use.

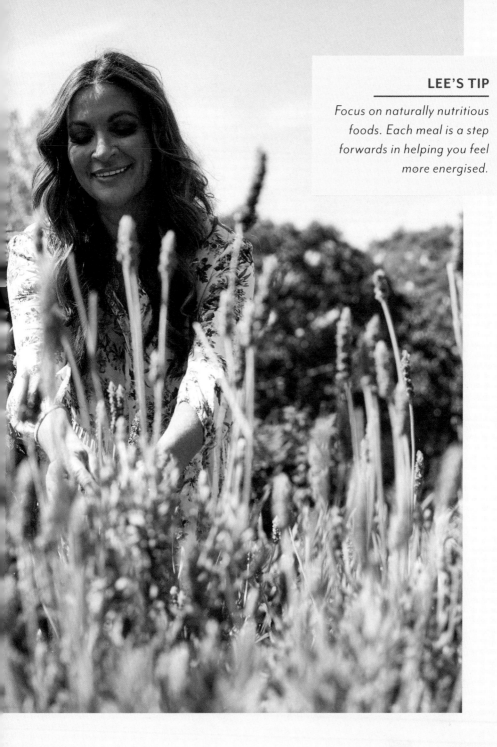

LEE'S TIP

Focus on naturally nutritious foods. Each meal is a step forwards in helping you feel more energised.

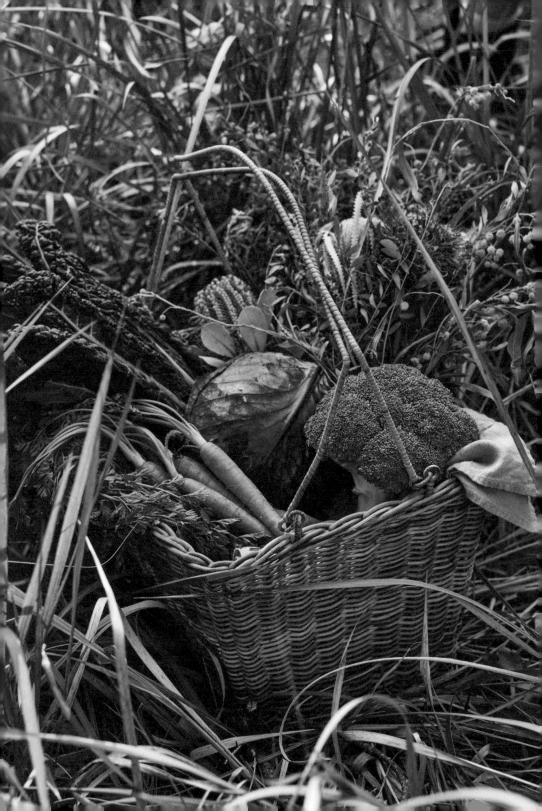

A low-histamine diet is a game-changer and kind to your system. It helps ease your symptoms and promote a more comfortable restorative experience.

Dietary changes: why a low-histamine diet works for Long Covid

As the first step, I recommend following an anti-inflammatory diet that promotes your cardiovascular and metabolic health while addressing the inflammation caused by COVID-19. This diet includes foods such as broccoli, garlic, blueberries and legumes, and incorporates ginger tea. Cooking with spices such as turmeric, celery seed, fennel and rosemary further enhances the food's anti-inflammatory effects. As the inflammatory processes subside, emphasising a fresh, low-histamine, wholefood, eating-with-the-seasons approach helps you build physical resilience and reduce your likelihood of future infections.

The first place to target your immunity is through your gut, where 70–80 per cent of your immune tissue resides. Because your gut is often the first entry point for pathogens, you want to ensure you have a good amount of gut flora to prevent pathogens and infections from being absorbed into your body through the gut lining.[70]

By consuming an anti-inflammatory diet and eating lots of fibre from fruit, vegetables and whole grains, you'll be on your way to supporting your gut. Prioritise foods and spices that reduce inflammation: think omega-3-rich salmon and fibre-rich flaxseeds (linseeds).

Because the gut and immune system are linked, a diet that supports healthy gut and immune function is full of prebiotics, probiotics and synbiotics. Including a synbiotic supplement is essential, alongside

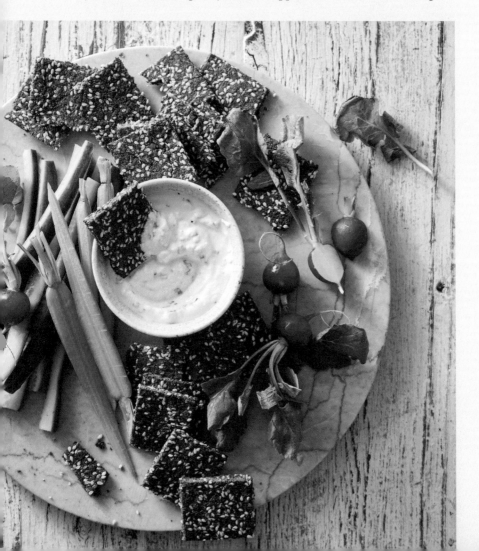

prebiotic-rich foods such as onion, chicory and asparagus. You can also incorporate prebiotic spices such as turmeric, ginger, rosemary and oregano to enhance your gut health. By focusing on these aspects, you'll optimise your gut microbiota and bolster your immune system as you recover from Long Covid.

Emerging evidence implies that probiotics may diminish your general susceptibility to infectious agents. More specifically, using probiotics may manipulate your intestinal microbiota and, in turn, modulate the immune system and its inflammatory responses.

TIPS TO HELP DIGESTION WHEN EATING	
Take your time.	Give your gut enough time to digest by not rushing through meals. Give yourself at least 30 minutes to eat, allowing for a more relaxed digestion process and minimising stress on your gut.
Chew thoroughly.	Remember, digestion begins in the mouth. Chew your food until it reaches a semi-liquid consistency. You'll make it easier for your gut to break down the food, reducing the strain on your digestive system.
Sit down and prioritise relaxation.	Instead of standing, take a seated position while you eat. Standing can trigger the fight-or-flight response, signalling danger to your body. Sitting down creates a sense of safety, enabling your body to focus on digestion and healing.
Gentle abdominal massage before meals.	If you experience digestive issues, try gently massaging your abdomen before eating. This practice helps to relax your abdominal muscles and encourages your body to shift into the parasympathetic mode, which promotes rest, healing and optimal digestion.
Have a smoothie.	Try including my Long Covid 'Medicinal' Recovery Smoothie (see page 191) in your daily diet to ensure a robust intake of anti-inflammatory nutrients and plant foods.

If you have Long Covid, a low-histamine diet can potentially help reduce any symptoms related to histamine intolerance or MCAS. During Long Covid, your immune system and inflammatory response may be dysregulated, leading your body to overproduce or impair the breakdown of histamine. This can result in headaches, itching, hives, flushes and gastrointestinal issues.

By following a low-histamine diet, you'll limit your intake of histamine-rich foods and foods that trigger the release of histamine. This can help reduce the overall histamine load in your body and alleviate symptoms of histamine intolerance.

Some foods that are high in histamine or trigger histamine release can also have pro-inflammatory effects, which can further exacerbate inflammation and immune dysfunction in your body. By avoiding these foods, you may experience less overall inflammation and less severe symptoms.

High levels of histamine can contribute to chronic inflammation in the body. By following a low-histamine diet, you'll be reducing your intake of histamine-rich foods that can contribute to inflammation, and you may experience less inflammation overall and an improvement of Long Covid symptoms.

Histamine is involved in the immune response – high levels of histamine can contribute to immune system dysfunction. By reducing your histamine intake, you'll be supporting your immune system, reducing your risk of infections.

Histamine intolerance can cause gastrointestinal symptoms including bloating, diarrhoea and abdominal pain. By reducing your histamine intake, you may see an improvement in your symptoms.

Histamine is also involved in the sleep-wake cycle, and high levels of histamine can contribute to difficulty sleeping or staying asleep. With a low-histamine diet, you'll improve your sleep quality and reduce fatigue. Histamine is a known trigger for headaches, which many long-haulers experience. By following a low-histamine diet, you may be able to reduce your headaches.

I found that reducing my intake of histamine-rich foods has helped to mitigate the impacts of MCAS and Long Covid significantly.[71] Cutting down sugar, and eliminating alcohol, food preservatives and additives, also contributed to my improvement.

While individual tolerances may vary, what follows is a snapshot of foods typically recommended on a low-histamine diet.

In managing histamine intolerance, your long-term goal is to support the proper functioning of your body's histamine pathways. This involves reducing mast cell over-reactivity, which is responsible for releasing excessive histamine. By addressing mast cell activation and minimising histamine triggers, you can begin to gradually reintroduce a wider variety of foods over time. This process requires an individualised approach, such as following a low-histamine diet, incorporating gut-healing protocols, and identifying and addressing the underlying factors contributing to histamine intolerance. But it is possible to restore balance to your histamine pathways and improve your tolerance to a greater range of foods.

When it comes to histamine content, certain foods have a dual nature. While they may contain higher levels of histamine, they also provide valuable compounds such as quercetin that have histamine-lowering properties. Quercetin is a flavonoid with anti-inflammatory and antioxidant effects. It acts as a natural antihistamine by inhibiting the release of histamine from mast cells and reducing the activity of histamine receptors.

If you have a histamine intolerance, by consuming foods that contain both histamine and quercetin you can potentially benefit from the balancing effect of these compounds. Citrus fruits, onions, garlic, berries, apples, parsley and capers, for example, not only provide important nutrients but also contribute to histamine regulation because they contain quercetin.

Because the impact of these foods can vary from person to person, you should take your individual tolerance level into consideration. If you have a severe histamine intolerance, you may still need to avoid high-histamine foods altogether, even if they contain histamine-lowering quercetin. Experimentation and personal observation are key to determining which foods you can tolerate and are beneficial for your specific needs.

Incorporating quercetin-rich foods into the diet, alongside a comprehensive approach to managing histamine intolerance, can potentially help to reduce your symptoms and improve overall well-being. I suggest working with a healthcare professional or registered dietitian experienced in histamine intolerance to create an individualised plan that considers your specific sensitivities and dietary requirements.

Stay positive! Each day is an opportunity for you to rebuild, evolve and move forward. Your choices, actions and resilience define the narrative of your life.

Meal planner

Here's your weekly meal planner designed specifically for you. It includes diverse and nutritious low-histamine recipes to support your recovery. Look for comforting options such as Maple Macadamia Granola and Coconut Cornflakes, as well as creative dishes like Rainbow Rice Paper Rolls and White Fish Corn Tortillas with Mango Salsa. Each recipe is thoughtfully

	MONDAY	TUESDAY	WEDNESDAY
Self-care	Listen to a guided meditation	Journal	Practise deep breathing exercise
Supplements			
Breakfast	Maple macadamia granola (p. 187)	Passionfruit & peach chia pudding (p. 189)	Sautéed greens breakfast bowl (egg optional) (p. 189)
Lunch	Warm asparagus salad (p. 197)	Pumpkin & quinoa soup (p. 198)	Hemp-crusted chicken & broccoli Buddha bowl (p. 201)
Dinner	Roasted capsicum pasta (p. 209)	White fish corn tortillas with mango salsa (p. 211)	Roasted pork fillet with kale & apple slaw (p. 213)
Snacks	White chocolate bark with blackcurrants & macadamia (p. 221)	Rosemary potato crisps (p. 221)	Roasted spiced macadamias & pecans (p. 223)

crafted to be full of flavour and provide the necessary nutrients to aid your recovery. Alongside these healing recipes are deep breathing exercises, journalling prompts and meditation sessions, which you can incorporate into your weekly routine. These practices are designed to nourish your mind and spirit along with your body.

THURSDAY	FRIDAY	SATURDAY	SUNDAY
Body scan meditation	Practise self-massage	Engage with nature, feel the ground beneath your feet	Write down three things you're grateful for
Dragon fruit & berry bowl (p. 191)	Coconut cornflakes (p. 193)	Mini veggie breakfast tarts (p. 195)	Long covid 'medicinal' recovery smoothie (p. 191)
Ginger salmon rice bowl (p. 203)	Minty beef–stuffed capsicums (p. 199)	Whipped ricotta & radish rice cakes (p. 207)	Rainbow rice paper rolls (p. 205)
Pesto chicken with cauliflower rice (p. 214)	Vegetarian gnocchi soup (p. 215)	Roasted cabbage with carrot purée & herb oil (p. 217)	Turkey, dried blueberry & quinoa-stuffed zucchini (p. 219)
Blueberry and basil smoothie bites (p. 223)	Ricotta rice cakes with passionfruit & honey (p. 226)	Air-fryer zucchini fries (p. 227)	Coconut, cranberry & macadamia slice (p. 225)

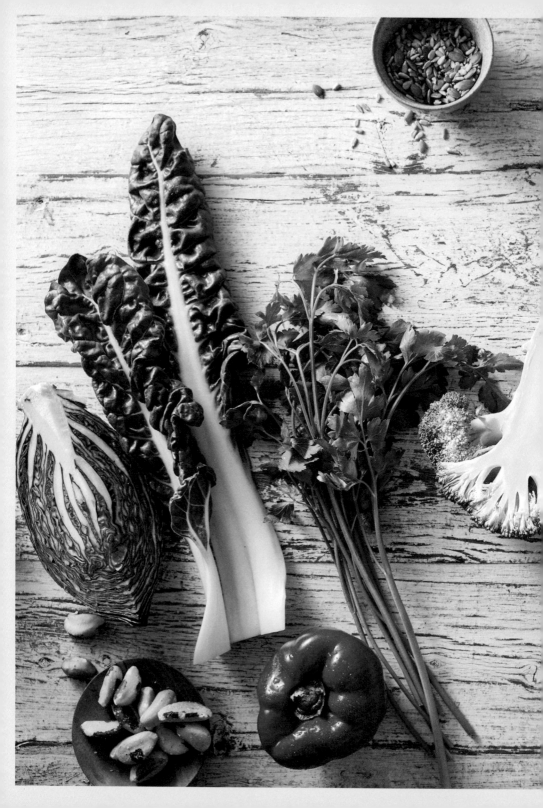

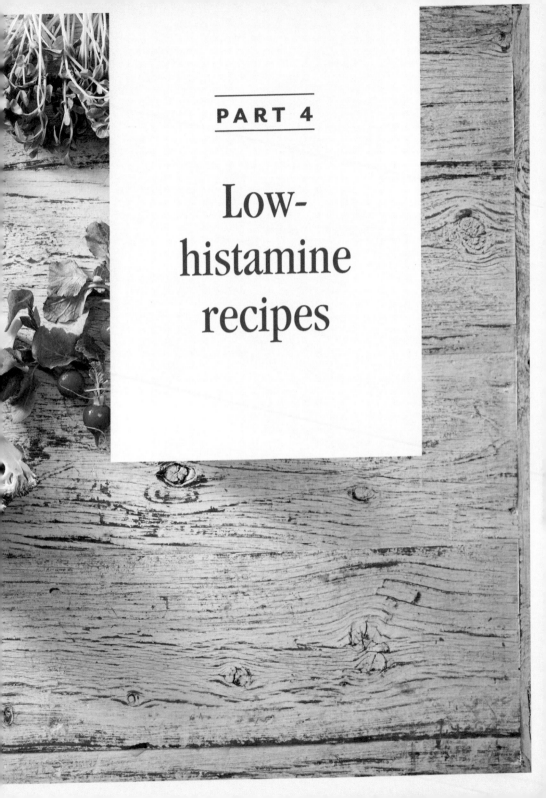

PART 4

Low-histamine recipes

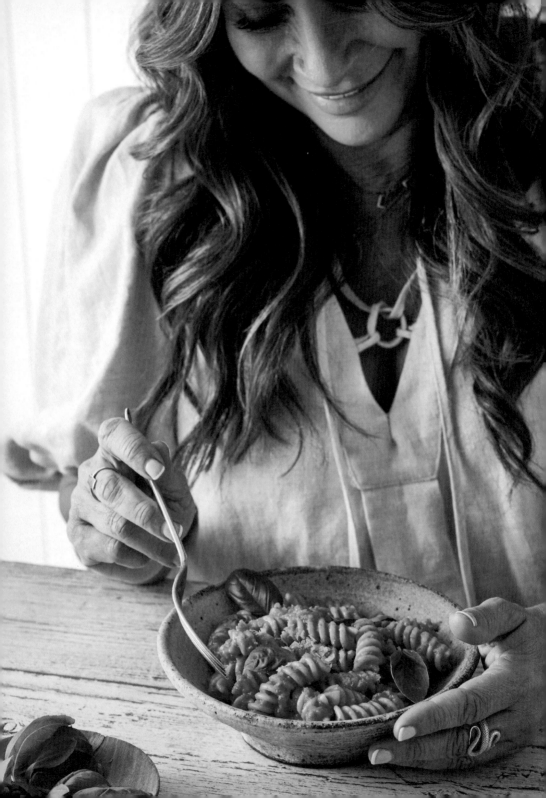

*Savour every bite of these
recipes, they will provide joy
and nourishment!*

Recipes

In this collection of 30 carefully crafted recipes, I invite you to embark on a culinary journey designed specifically for Long Covid. These recipes have been thoughtfully curated to be low in histamines while supporting your well-being and nourishing you as you navigate towards recovery.

Starting with enticing breakfast options, such as the delightful Maple Macadamia Granola and the refreshing Dragon Fruit & Berry Bowl, you'll kick-start your day with flavours that awaken your senses and provide a gentle boost of energy. For those seeking a comforting and nutritious morning meal, the Sautéed Greens Breakfast Bowl and Long Covid 'Medicinal' Recovery Smoothie are sure to satisfy your cravings.

My lunch recipes offer a mix of vibrant salads, hearty soups and satisfying bowls. Indulge in the aromatic Warm Asparagus Salad or the wholesome goodness of Pumpkin & Quinoa Soup. If a protein-packed option is your preference, the Hemp-crusted Chicken & Broccoli Buddha Bowl is a perfect choice.

As the day transitions into dinner, from the comforting Roasted Capsicum Pasta to the tantalising White Fish Corn Tortillas with Mango Salsa, each dish is designed to bring joy to your evening meals. Explore the flavours of Roast Pork Fillet with Kale &

Apple Slaw or savour the fragrant Pesto Chicken with Cauliflower Rice. These recipes cater to a range of dietary preferences, including options like Vegetarian Gnocchi Soup for those seeking a wholesome vegetarian delight.

I haven't forgotten about the importance of satisfying snacks either. Indulge in treats like the decadent White Chocolate Bark with Blackcurrants & Macadamia, or enjoy the crispy and savoury Rosemary Potato Crisps. For a quick and nutritious bite, try the Blueberry & Basil Smoothie Bites or the Ricotta Rice Cakes with Passionfruit & Honey.

To complement your meals, I've also included options like Rice Flour Bread with Chia & Flaxseed and Ginger, Turmeric & Sesame Crackers, which add a touch of homemade goodness.

These recipes are a testament to the belief that healing yourself can be nourishing and flavourful. Embrace these recipes as part of your journey towards wellness, savouring every bite and finding joy in the nourishment they provide.

Please note that individual sensitivities may vary, so it's important to consult with a healthcare professional or registered dietitian to ensure these recipes align with your specific needs and dietary requirements. Let these recipes be your companion as you unmask the possibilities of delicious, low-histamine meals on your path to recovery.

✳ A NOTE ABOUT THE MEASUREMENTS ✳

✦ Please note that the cup and spoon measures in these recipes are based on Australian sizes. (The USA and UK use 15 ml tablespoon measures.)

✦ 1 cup = 250 ml/9 fl oz

✦ 1 tablespoon = 20 ml/½ fl oz

✳ A GUIDE TO SYMBOLS ✳

gf gluten free

wf wheat free

df dairy free

sf sugar free

vt vegetarian

ve vegan

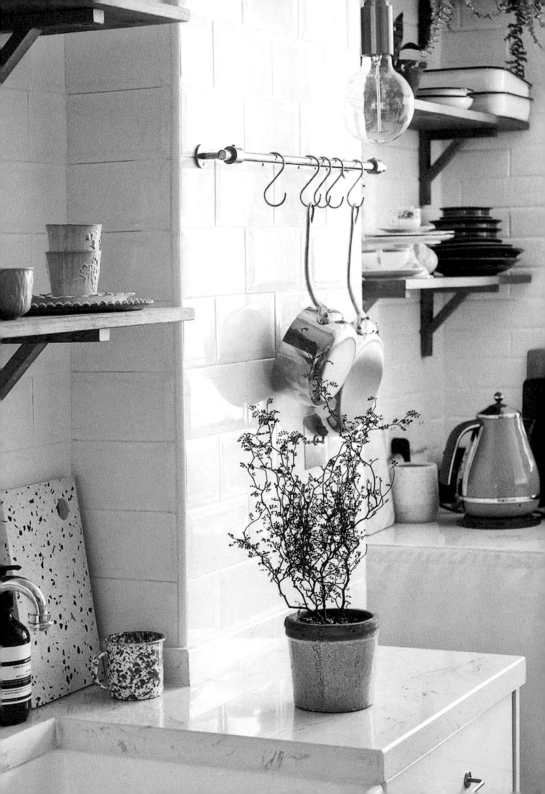

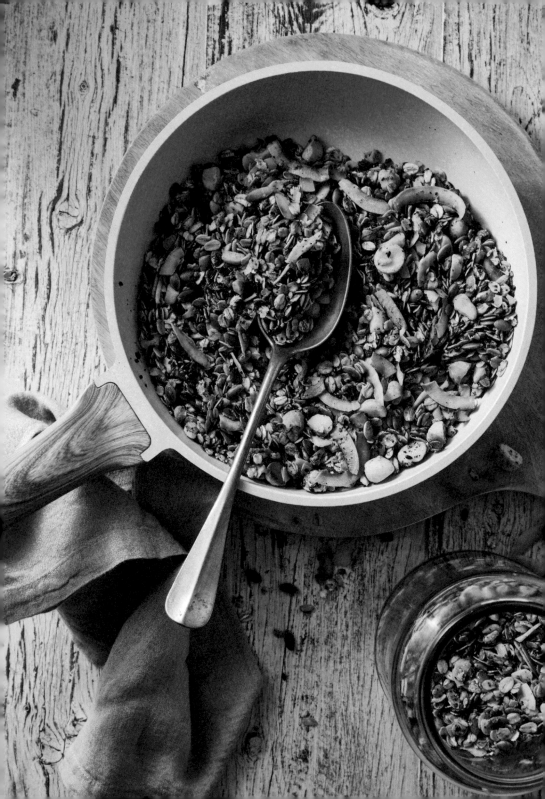

Maple macadamia granola

Serves 8   gf   wf   df   sf   vt   ve

2 cups rolled oats

½ cup macadamias, roughly chopped

¼ cup flaxseeds (linseeds)

¼ cup pumpkin seeds

¼ cup coconut flakes

½ tsp salt

2 tbsp coconut oil

2 tbsp maple syrup

Coconut milk, to serve

Fresh blueberries, to serve

1. Heat a large frying pan over medium–low heat. Add the oats, macadamias, seeds, coconut flakes and salt. Stir until golden, then pour coconut oil over the oat mixture and remove from heat.

2. Drizzle maple syrup over and stir thoroughly. Let the mixture cool to room temperature.

3. Serve the granola with coconut milk and fresh blueberries. Store the rest in an airtight jar.

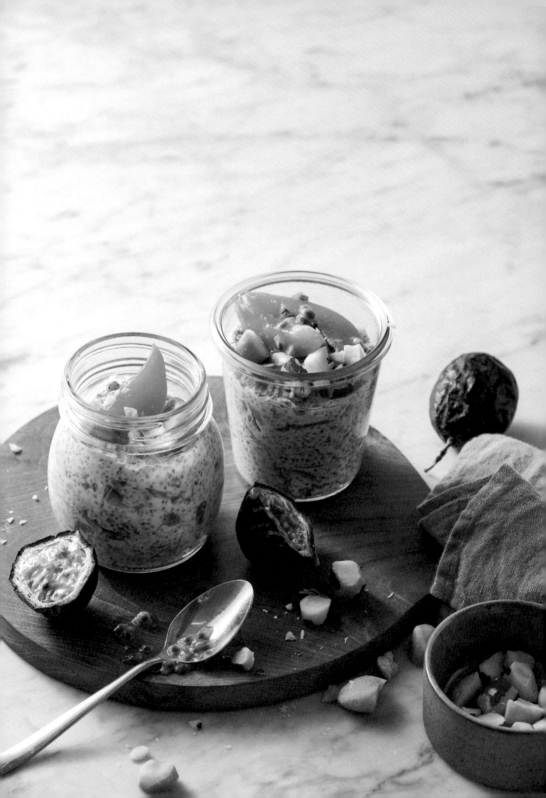

Passionfruit & peach chia pudding

Serves 2   gf   wf   df   sf   vt   ve

¼ cup chia seeds

1 cup coconut milk

2 tbsp maple syrup

1 passionfruit, pulp only

½ peach, diced

1 passionfruit, pulp only, to serve

¼ cup brazil nuts, roughly chopped, to serve

1. Combine the chia seeds, coconut milk, maple syrup, passionfruit pulp and peach in a small bowl. Divide the mixture between 2 x 1-cup glasses or Mason jars. Cover and leave in the fridge overnight to set.

2. In the morning, serve with passionfruit pulp and a sprinkle of brazil nuts.

Sautéed greens breakfast bowl

Serves 1   gf   wf   df   sf   vt   ve

2 tbsp extra-virgin olive oil, plus extra to serve

½ small brown onion, diced finely

½ cup hazelnuts or macadamias roughly chopped (optional)

Salt, to taste

1 cup asparagus, chopped

2 cups kale, chopped

1 tbsp sweet paprika, ground

½ cup parsley, roughly chopped

2 tbsp pomegranate seeds

1 egg, boiled, peeled and halved (optional)

Handful pea shoots, to serve

1. Heat the oil in a large frying pan (skillet) over medium heat. Add the onion, stirring frequently, and cook until softened and fragrant, about 3–5 minutes.

2. Add the hazelnuts and a pinch of salt, then stir in the asparagus, kale and paprika.

3. Once the kale has wilted, remove from the heat. Add the parsley and pomegranate seeds, stirring well.

4. Serve in a large bowl with the boiled egg, pea shoots, a sprinkle of salt and a drizzle of olive oil. Enjoy while warm!

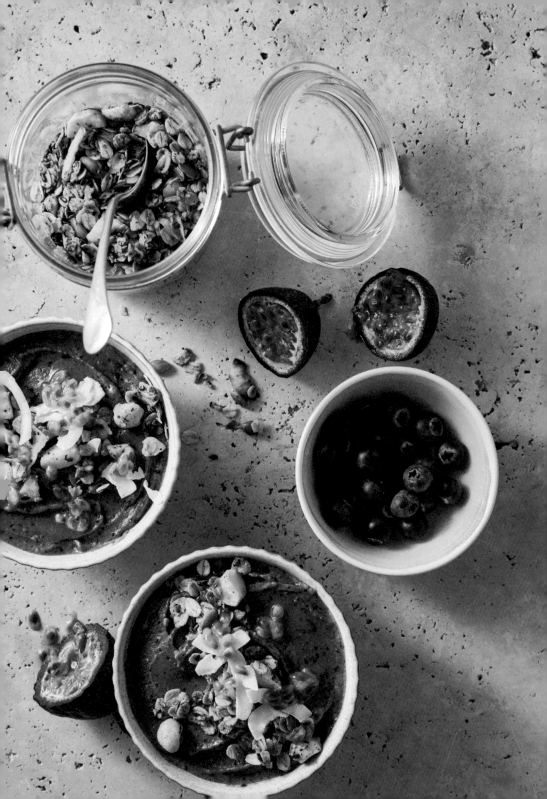

Dragon fruit & berry bowl

Serves 3   gf wf df sf vt ve

2 cups frozen
dragon fruit (pitaya) chunks

1 cup frozen
mango, chopped

1 cup frozen blueberries

1 frozen banana

1 tbsp flaxseed (linseed) meal

1 tbsp Love Your Gut Synbiotic

1 cup canned
coconut milk

TOPPINGS

Coconut flakes

Maple Macadamia
Granola (see page 187)

Fresh blueberries

Passionfruit

1. Place all the frozen ingredients plus the flaxseed meal, Love Your Gut Synbiotic and coconut milk in a high-speed blender and whiz until creamy and smooth.

2. Add a little more milk to thin the smoothie, if necessary.

3. Scoop into two serving bowls and top with coconut flakes, granola, blueberries and passionfruit.

Long Covid 'medicinal' recovery smoothie

Serves 1   gf wf df sf vt ve

1 cup coconut water

2 celery stalks

½ apple

½ cucumber

½ banana

½ cup frozen mango

¼ cup blueberries

Handful rocket

Handful kale

1 scoop NAC powder

1 tsp Love Your Gut Synbiotic[1] or
Love Your Gut powder[2]

1 tsp vitamin C powder

½ tsp ginger (optional)

1 quercetin tablet

1–2 ice cubes

1. Place all ingredients in a high-speed blender and blend until smooth.

[1] superchargeyourgut.com

[2] superchargeyourgut.com

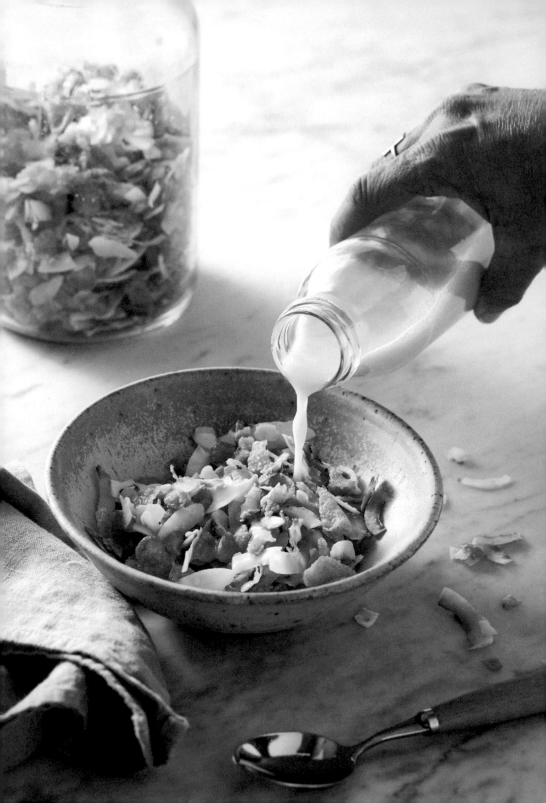

Coconut cornflakes

Serves 4   gf   wf   df   sf   vt

2 tbsp coconut oil

2 cups coconut flakes

2 cups organic cornflakes

1 tbsp honey or maple syrup

½ tsp salt

Coconut, goat's or sheep's milk, to serve

1. Heat 1 tbsp coconut oil in a large pan over medium–high heat. Add the coconut flakes and toast until golden and crunchy.

2. Remove from heat and add the cornflakes, honey, salt and remaining oil. Stir thoroughly, set aside and cool to room temperature.

3. Serve with coconut, goat's or sheep's milk. Store the remaining cornflakes in an airtight container or jar.

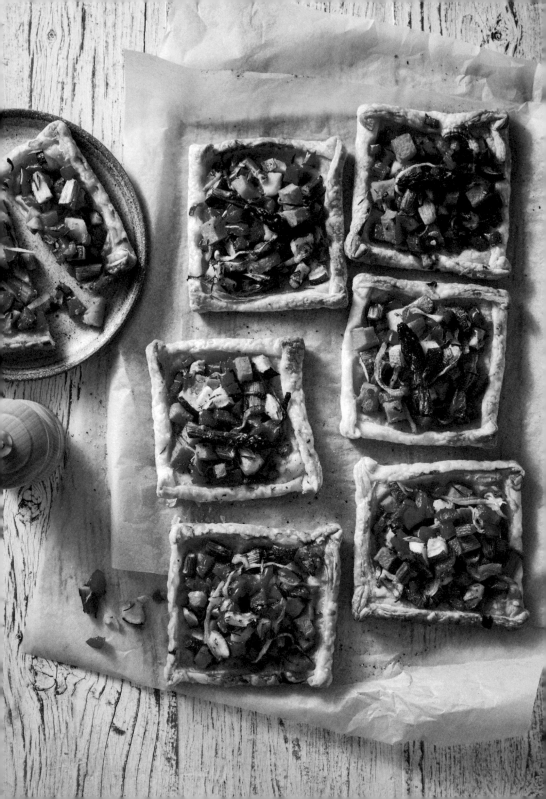

Mini veggie breakfast tarts

Makes 8 tarts   gf   wf   df   sf   vt   ve

1 sheet frozen puff pastry

Olive oil spray

100 g (3½ oz) butternut pumpkin, diced

4 asparagus spears, diced

½ zucchini, diced

1 red capsicum, diced

½ brown onion, thinly sliced

2 sprigs fresh rosemary, chopped

2 tbsp extra-virgin olive oil

Salt, to taste

1. Preheat the oven to 200°C (400°F). Line 2 large baking trays with paper.

2. Once the pastry has slightly defrosted, cut into 8 equal squares and place on the prepared baking trays. Fold in the edges to make a ½ cm (¼ inch) border. Lightly spray with oil.

3. Steam the pumpkin, asparagus and zucchini over boiling water until just tender.

4. Transfer vegetables to a large bowl and combine with the capsicum, onion, rosemary, olive oil and salt.

5. Scoop the vegetable mixture into each tart case. Place the tray into the oven and bake for 15–20 minutes or until the pastry is golden. Serve warm!

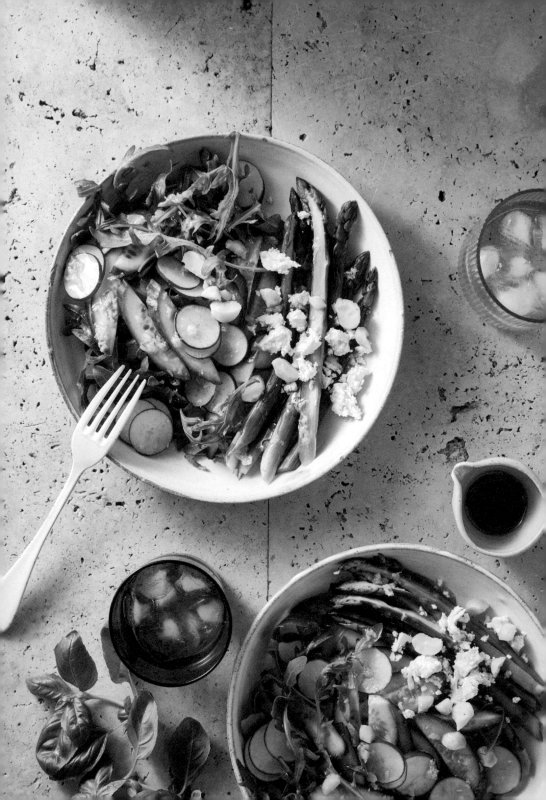

Warm asparagus salad

Serves 2   gf wf df sf vt ve

250 g (9 oz) asparagus, halved

100 g (3½ oz) rocket

1 cucumber, thinly sliced

4 small red radishes, thinly sliced

Handful fresh basil

⅓ cup macadamias, roughly chopped

Crumbled feta, to serve (optional)

DRESSING

4 tbsp extra-virgin olive oil

1 tsp apple cider vinegar

1 tsp garlic, grated

1 tsp ginger, grated

Salt, to taste

1. Steam the asparagus over boiling water until tender. Drain and set aside.

2. To make the dressing, combine all the ingredients in a small bowl. In a large bowl, toss the salad ingredients together then drizzle the dressing over.

3. Top with crumbled feta if desired and enjoy!

Pumpkin & quinoa soup

Serves 4   gf   wf   df   sf   vt   ve

500 g (1 lb 2 oz) butternut pumpkin, peeled, seeded and chopped into cubes

2 red capsicums, chopped into cubes

2 garlic cloves, sliced

4 tbsp extra-virgin olive oil

1 brown onion, diced

2 celery stalks, diced

1 knob ginger, grated

Salt

4 cups vegetable broth

2 cups water

2 tbsp sweet paprika

1 tsp cumin

½ tsp dried thyme

1 cup quinoa, rinsed

100 g (3½ oz) kale, roughly chopped

Rice Flour Bread with Chia & Flaxseed (see page 229), to serve (optional)

1. Preheat the oven to 180°C (350°F).

2. Toss the pumpkin, capsicums and garlic in 2 tbsp olive oil and place on a lined baking tray. Bake in the oven for 20–30 minutes until roasted.

3. Meanwhile, heat another 2 tbsp olive oil in a large stockpot over medium–high heat. Add the onion and sauté for 7–8 minutes or until translucent and fragrant.

4. Add the celery, ginger and a pinch of salt then cook for 3–5 minutes, stirring frequently. Add the roasted pumpkin mixture, broth and water. Season with the paprika, cumin and thyme. Increase the heat and bring to a light boil.

5. Once boiling, add the quinoa, reduce heat to a light simmer and cover. Cook for about 20 minutes or until the quinoa is fluffy. In the last 5 minutes of cooking, add the kale and season with salt.

6. Serve while still warm, with a slice of rice flour bread (optional).

Minty beef-stuffed capsicums

Serves 1   gf wf df sf

2 tbsp extra-virgin olive oil

½ brown onion, finely diced

120 g (4¼ oz) beef mince

Salt, to taste

Large handful fresh mint leaves, chopped

1 tsp fresh or dried rosemary

1 tsp ground coriander

1 tsp sweet paprika

½ small zucchini, finely diced

½ cup flaked almonds, plus extra to serve

1 red or green capsicum, halved lengthwise, core and seeds removed

Nutritional yeast flakes

Handful rocket, to serve

1. Preheat the oven to 200°C (400°F).
2. Heat 1 tbsp olive oil in a large frying pan (skillet) over medium heat and cook the onion for 2–5 minutes.
3. Add the mince, season with salt and then cook, stirring frequently, for 5 minutes or until the mince is cooked through. Stir in the mint, rosemary, ground coriander, paprika, zucchini and flaked almonds. Turn down the heat and simmer for about 5 minutes.
4. Place the capsicum halves cut side up in a lined baking dish and drizzle with the remaining oil.
5. Spoon the mince mixture into each capsicum half and sprinkle with some nutritional yeast flakes.
6. Bake until the capsicums are tender, about 20–25 minutes.
7. Remove from the oven and serve with rocket and flaked almonds.

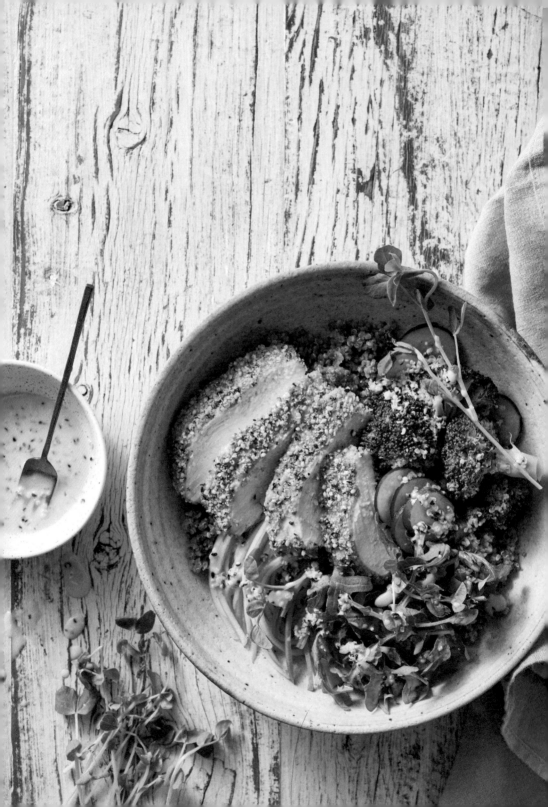

Hemp-crusted chicken & broccoli Buddha bowl

Serves 1   gf wf df sf

2 tbsp almond meal

2 tbsp hemp seeds

½ tsp garlic powder

½ tsp sweet paprika

Salt and pepper, to taste

1 tbsp tapioca starch, blended with
   3 tsp water

1 skinless chicken breast

1 cup quinoa, cooked

Small handful pea shoots, to serve

SALAD

¼ head broccoli, steamed

1 carrot, sliced using a vegetable
   peeler

1 cucumber, peeled and sliced

2 radishes, thinly sliced

Handful rocket

DRESSING

2 tbsp extra-virgin olive oil

2 tbsp water

1 tsp apple cider vinegar

1 tbsp hemp seeds

1 tbsp tahini

½ tsp grated ginger

Salt

1. Preheat the oven to 200°C (400°F).

2. Combine the almond meal, hemp seeds, garlic powder, paprika, salt and pepper in a shallow dish. In a separate shallow dish, add the tapioca mixture. Place the tapioca dish, hemp dish and a lined baking tray in a row.

3. Dip the chicken breast first in the tapioca then the hemp mixture. Place on the baking tray. Bake for 15–20 minutes before removing and slicing into strips.

4. To make the dressing, combine all the ingredients together in a small bowl.

5. To make the salad, add the quinoa to a large serving bowl, then add all the salad ingredients in individual piles. Top with the chicken, drizzle dressing generously over and scatter some pea shoots to serve.

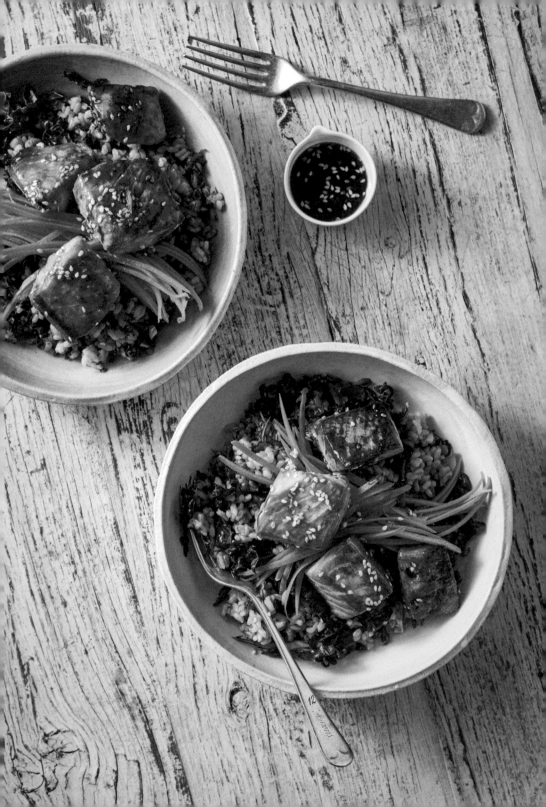

Ginger salmon rice bowl

Serves 2   gf wf df sf

2 tsp extra-virgin olive oil, divided

2 salmon fillets, cut into chunks

1 cup red cabbage, shredded

1 small bunch kale, shredded

2 cups cooked brown rice

¼ cup fresh basil, chopped

1 carrot, grated

MARINADE

2.5 cm (1 inch) piece fresh ginger, grated

4 tbsp sesame oil

4 tbsp tamari

2 tbsp honey

1 tbsp sesame seeds

1. To make the marinade, whisk all the ingredients together in a small bowl.

2. Heat 1½ tsp olive oil in a large frying pan (skillet) over medium–high heat. Add the salmon chunks and brown on all sides for 2–3 minutes.

3. Lower the heat and stir in the marinade, reserving a small amount to dress the salad. Simmer for a further 3–4 minutes or until the salmon is cooked through. Remove from heat and set aside.

4. Using the same pan, cook the red cabbage and kale in 1 tsp olive oil, then set aside.

5. In a large mixing bowl, combine the cooked brown rice, kale and cabbage. Add the basil then pour a little bit of the reserved marinade over. Toss well.

6. Divide the rice mixture into two serving bowls. Top with carrot and salmon and a drizzle of the remaining marinade. Enjoy while warm!

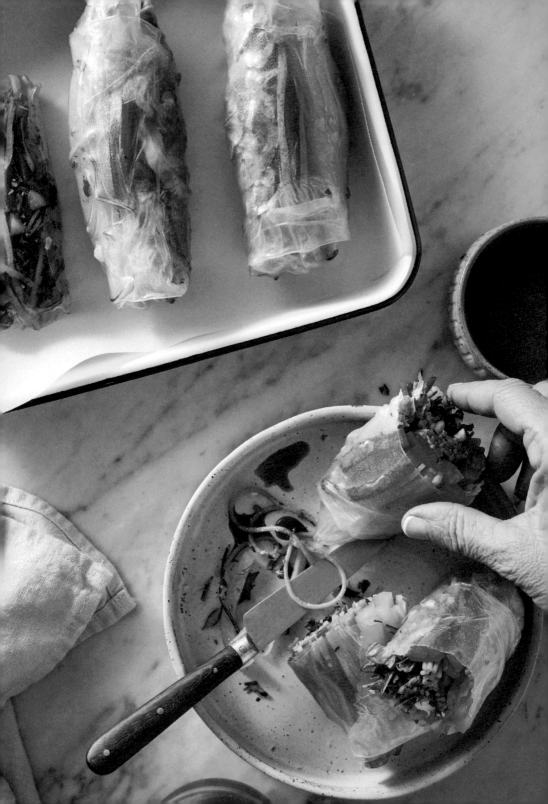

Rainbow rice paper rolls

Makes 10 rolls   gf   wf   df   sf   vt

10 rice paper sheets

FILLING

6 small organic romaine or gem
 lettuce leaves, finely sliced

100 g (3½ oz) brown rice vermicelli,
 blanched and cooled

1 cucumber, sliced into thin batons

1 carrot, sliced into thin batons

1 red capsicum, sliced into thin
 batons

1 yellow capsicum, sliced into thin
 batons

¼ red cabbage, shredded

½ bunch fresh mint, finely chopped

½ bunch fresh coriander, finely
 chopped

½ cup macadamias, finely chopped

DIPPING SAUCE

½ cup water

2 tbsp tamari

1 tbsp honey

1 tbsp sweet paprika

½ tbsp almond or nut butter

2.5 cm (1 inch) piece fresh ginger,
 grated

1 garlic clove, minced

1. To make the dipping sauce, whisk the ingredients together thoroughly in a small
    bowl then transfer to a dipping dish.
2. Prepare a rolling station with all the filling ingredients, rice paper sheets, a damp
    chopping board and a large shallow dish filled with warm water.
3. Soak one rice paper sheet in warm water, lay it on the chopping board and start
    to layer vegetables on one side. Start with a lettuce leaf then add some noodles,
    a small handful of each veggie and herb, and a sprinkle of macadamias.
4. Gently roll the rice paper over the mixture away from you, folding the sides
    inward as you roll until the end. Repeat with the other rice paper sheets.
5. Cut the rolls into half and serve with the dipping sauce.

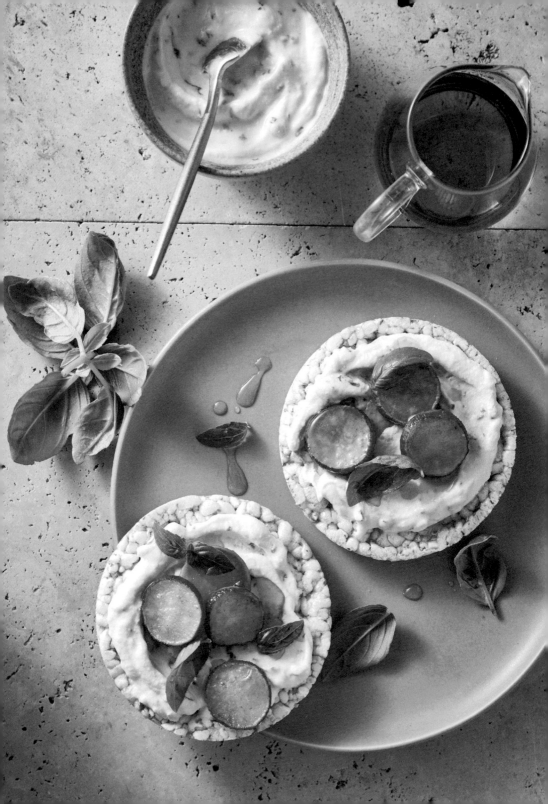

Whipped ricotta & radish rice cakes

Serves 2   gf   wf   df   sf   vt

6 small radishes, halved

3 tbsp extra-virgin olive oil

2 tbsp maple syrup

1 tsp cumin

1 container (300 g/10½ oz) ricotta cheese

1 bunch basil leaves

2 tbsp water

1 tsp apple cider vinegar

1 garlic clove, chopped

Salt, to taste

4 puffed rice cakes

1. Preheat the oven to 180°C (350°F) and line a baking tray with paper.

2. Toss the radishes with 1 tbsp olive oil, 1 tbsp maple syrup and all the cumin. Spread evenly across the baking tray. Bake for 10–15 minutes or until the radishes are just cooked. Set aside.

3. Meanwhile, add the ricotta, remaining maple syrup, half the basil leaves, water, apple cider vinegar, garlic and salt to a food processor. Blend until whipped and creamy.

4. Spread the whipped ricotta generously over each rice cake, then top with roasted radishes, torn basil leaves, a pinch of salt and a drizzle of olive oil.

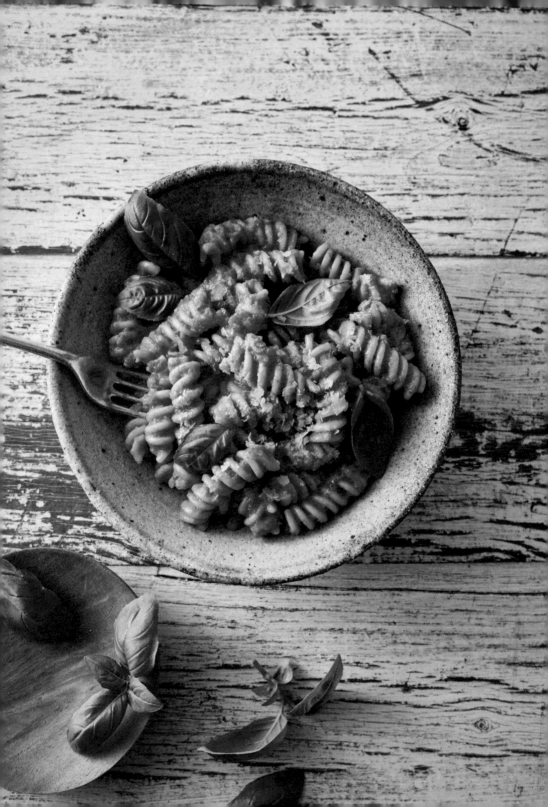

Roasted capsicum pasta

Serves 4   gf wf df sf vt ve

2 red capsicums

2 yellow capsicums

3 tbsp extra-virgin olive oil

Salt, to taste

350 g (12 oz) spelt or rice pasta of your choice

1 brown onion, finely diced

4 garlic cloves, finely diced

4 tbsp nutritional yeast flakes, plus extra to serve

½ cup coconut milk

Fresh basil leaves, to serve

1. Preheat the oven to 220°C (430°F).

2. Place the whole capsicums on a lined baking tray. Season with 2 tbsp olive oil and a pinch of salt.

3. Roast for approximately 30 minutes, then remove from oven and cover in foil. Leave under the foil for 10 minutes before removing the charred skin and seeds. Set aside.

4. Add the pasta to boiling salted water and cook according to the packet instructions. Drain and set aside.

5. Meanwhile, heat 1 tbsp olive oil in a large pan. Sauté the onion and garlic until soft and fragrant, about 3–5 minutes.

6. Transfer the onion mixture, roasted capsicum, yeast flakes, coconut milk and salt to a food processor and blend until smooth. Return the capsicum sauce to the pan over low heat and gently bring to the boil.

7. Once boiling, turn down the heat and let the sauce simmer until it thickens.

8. Remove from heat and add the cooked pasta to the sauce, stirring well to combine. Serve with a sprinkle of yeast flakes and fresh basil.

Dinner

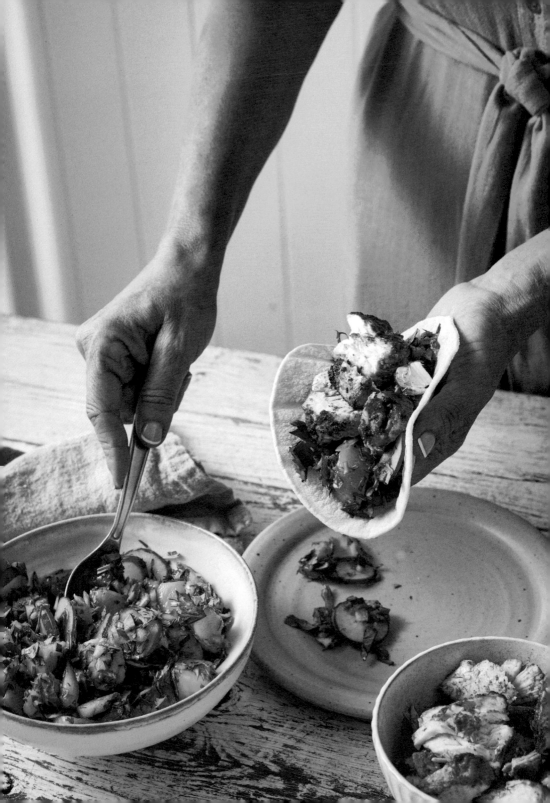

White fish corn tortillas with mango salsa

Serves 4   gf   wf   df   sf

2 tbsp extra-virgin olive oil, plus extra for frying

2 tbsp ground sweet paprika

1 tbsp ground cumin

2 garlic cloves, minced

Salt, to taste

4 fillets of firm white fish (cod or monk fish)

8 small corn tortillas

MANGO SALSA

2 mangoes, peeled and diced

¼ red cabbage, sliced

½ red onion, finely diced

4 radishes, sliced

1 bunch coriander, roughly chopped

2 tbsp extra-virgin olive oil

½ tbsp apple cider vinegar

Salt, to taste

1. Combine the olive oil, paprika, cumin, garlic and salt in a small bowl.

2. Rub the mixture thoroughly onto each fish fillet. Set aside.

3. To make the mango salsa, combine all the ingredients in a large mixing bowl and toss thoroughly. Set aside.

4. Heat some olive oil in a large frying pan (skillet) over medium–high heat. Add the fish fillets and cook for 3–5 minutes each side. Remove and let cool, then gently flake apart.

5. Prepare the tacos by filling each tortilla with a handful of fish and 2 scoops of salsa.

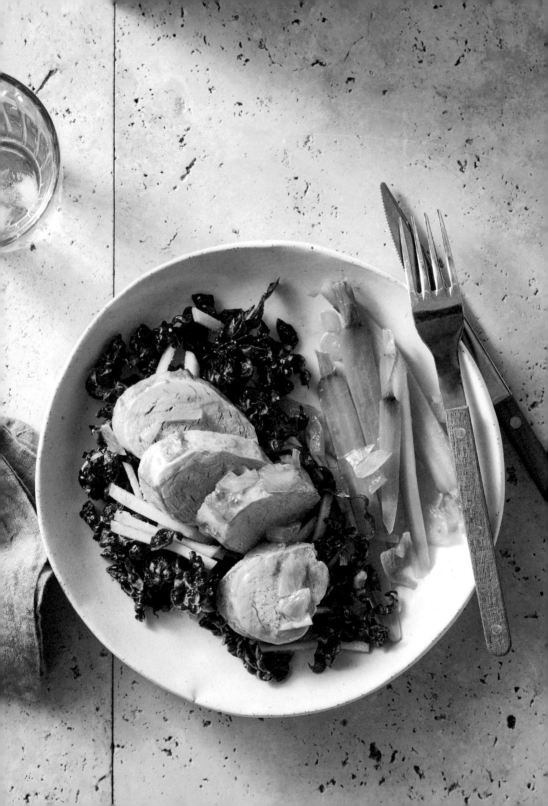

Roast pork fillet with kale & apple slaw

Serves 3–4   gf wf df sf

4 tbsp extra-virgin olive oil

1 pork tenderloin

1 bunch Dutch carrots, halved

1 brown onion, roughly chopped

Salt, to taste

1 bunch kale with stems removed, sliced thinly

1 granny smith (green) apple, cored and cut into thin matchsticks

¼ cup dried cranberries

¼ cup macadamias, roughly chopped

2 tbsp nutritional yeast flakes

1. Preheat the oven to 200°C (400°F).

2. Heat 1 tbsp olive oil in an ovenproof pan over high heat. Add the pork and sear on each side until golden, about 5 minutes.

3. Remove pan from heat then add the carrots and onion and 1 tbsp olive oil. Season generously with salt. Bake in the oven for 15–20 minutes or until cooked through.

4. Meanwhile, combine the kale, apple, cranberries, macadamias, yeast flakes and 2 tbsp olive oil in a large mixing bowl and toss to combine.

5. When the pork mixture is ready, remove from oven. Transfer the pork to a chopping board and let rest for 10 minutes. Slice the pork and serve on top of the kale and apple salad with the roasted carrots and onion alongside.

Dinner

Pesto chicken with cauliflower rice

Serves 4   gf   wf   df   sf

1 small head cauliflower,
roughly chopped

3 tbsp extra-virgin olive oil

4 boneless skinless chicken breasts,
cubed

Salt, to taste

3 tbsp water

1 cup fresh baby spinach leaves

2 large handfuls basil leaves, torn

PESTO

1 cup blanched almonds

2 garlic cloves, peeled

2 large handfuls fresh basil leaves

4 tbsp extra-virgin olive oil

1 tbsp apple cider vinegar

2 tbsp nutritional yeast flakes,
plus extra to serve

Pinch sea salt

1. To make the pesto, place the almonds in a food processor and blitz until fine. Add the garlic and pulse. Add the basil and blend again. Slowly drizzle in the olive oil until you have the desired consistency, then add the apple cider vinegar, yeast flakes and salt. Remove pesto from food processor and store in an airtight container or jar in the fridge (makes 1–2 cups).

2. After cleaning the food processor, add the cauliflower to the bowl and pulse until it resembles rice. Set aside.

3. Heat 2 tbsp olive oil in a large frying pan over medium–high heat. Season the chicken with salt then add to the pan. Sear on all sides for 8–10 minutes or until golden. Remove from pan and set aside.

4. Add 1 tbsp olive oil to the pan, then add the cauliflower rice. Sauté for about 3–5 minutes, stirring frequently.

5. Return the chicken to the pan and stir in ½ cup pesto and the water. Stir thoroughly to combine. Turn down the heat and simmer for 3–5 minutes.

6. Remove from heat and throw in the spinach and basil. Stir well until wilted.

7. Divide into portions and serve with a sprinkle of sea salt and yeast flakes.

Vegetarian gnocchi soup

Serves 4   gf   wf   df   sf   vt   ve

3 tbsp extra-virgin olive oil

2 celery stalks, chopped

2 carrots, grated

1 brown onion, finely diced

½ broccoli head, chopped

2 tbsp dried thyme

1 tsp ground cumin

1 tsp ground ginger

Salt, to taste

50 g (1¾ oz) butter

3 cups organic coconut milk

1 cup organic vegetable broth

1 packet (500 g/1 lb 2 oz) potato gnocchi

Small bunch kale with stems removed, roughly chopped

Nutritional yeast flakes, to serve

1. Heat the olive oil in a large stock pot over medium heat. Add the celery, and carrots and onion and sauté for about 3–5 minutes until the onions become translucent.

2. Add the broccoli, thyme, cumin, ginger and salt. Cook for a further 3–5 minutes or until the broccoli has softened, stirring occasionally.

3. Add the butter to the pan and stir well. Once the butter has melted, add in the coconut milk and vegetable broth. Bring to a soft boil then lower the heat to a simmer for 10–15 minutes.

4. Place the gnocchi in the pan and add the kale. Cook for 5–7 minutes or until the gnocchi is cooked through and the kale is wilted.

5. Serve with a sprinkle of salt and nutritional yeast flakes.

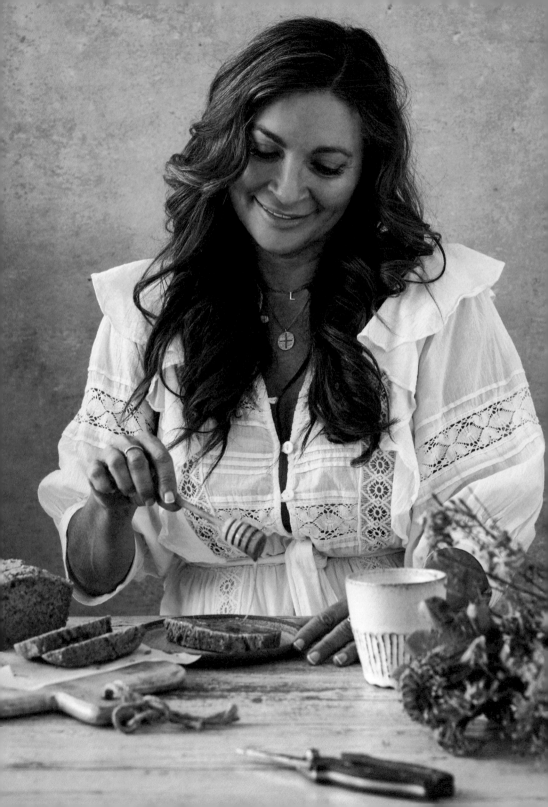

Roasted cabbage with carrot purée & herb oil

Serves 4–6   gf wf df sf vt

1 large green cabbage with outer leaves removed, cut into quarters

2 tbsp extra-virgin olive oil

1 tbsp garlic powder

Salt, to taste

CARROT PURÉE

4 large carrots, chopped into rounds or chunks

1 brown onion, peeled and cut into quarters

2 garlic cloves, peeled

2 tbsp extra-virgin olive oil

Salt, to taste

½ cup coconut milk

50 g (1¾ oz) butter, melted

HERB OIL

1 bunch fresh parsley

½ cup extra-virgin olive oil

2 tbsp apple cider vinegar

Salt, to taste

1. Preheat the oven to 200°C (400°F). Line two baking trays with baking paper.

2. Place the cabbage quarters flat onto one lined baking tray. Season with the olive oil, garlic powder and salt. Add to the top shelf of the oven and bake for 45 minutes or until golden and softened.

3. Meanwhile, place the carrots, onion and garlic on the other lined baking tray. Season with 1 tbsp olive oil and salt. Move the cabbage to the lower shelf and place the carrot mixture on the top shelf. Roast until the carrots are tender and browned, about 20 minutes.

4. Remove from oven and scoop the roasted carrot mixture into a food processor. Add the coconut milk, butter, remaining olive oil and salt. Blitz until smooth. Add more coconut milk for a thinner consistency if desired and set aside.

5. While the cabbage is still roasting, prepare the herb oil. Add all the ingredients to a blender and pulse until thoroughly blended. Pour into a sauce boat and set aside.

6. Reheat the carrot purée, if needed. Spoon 3 large tbsp onto each serving plate. Top with roasted cabbage and a drizzle of herb oil.

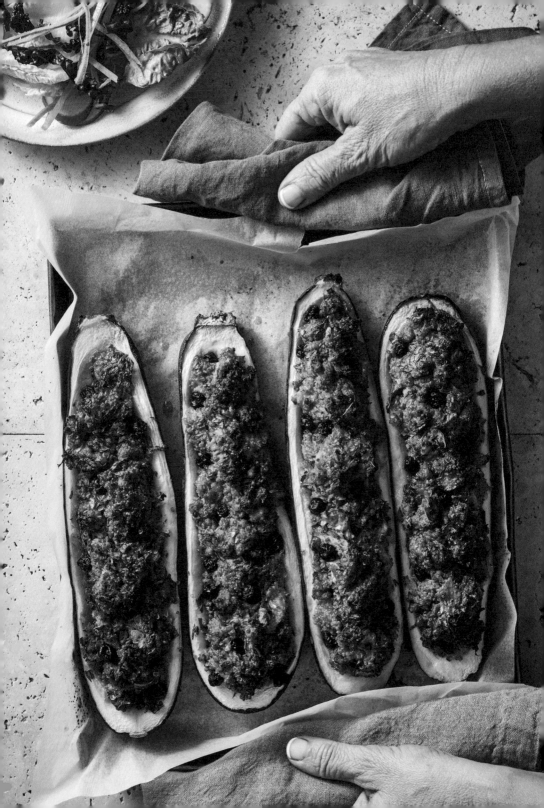

Turkey, dried blueberry & quinoa-stuffed zucchini

Serves 2   gf   wf   df   sf

2 large zucchini, halved lengthwise

4 tbsp extra-virgin olive oil

1 small brown onion, finely diced

1 garlic clove, minced

250 g (9 oz) turkey mince

1 tsp ground coriander

1 tsp ground cumin

1 tsp ground sweet paprika

½ tsp ground ginger

2 tbsp water

½ cup quinoa, cooked according to packet instructions

1 bunch fresh parsley, chopped

¼ cup dried blueberries

Salt, to taste

1. Preheat the oven to 200°C (400°F).

2. Carefully use a spoon to scoop out the zucchinl flesh without piercing the skin. Finely dice the zucchini flesh and set aside. Place the zucchini boats onto a lined baking tray.

3. Heat 1 tbsp olive oil in a large pan over medium–high heat. Add the onion and garlic and sauté for 5–6 minutes. Add the turkey mince and spices and stir thoroughly. Cook for 5–10 minutes or until turkey has browned.

4. Add the water to the pan, turn down to a simmer and stir in the cooked quinoa, parsley, dried blueberries and zucchini flesh. Cook for a further 3–5 minutes then remove pan from heat.

5. Scoop the turkey mixture evenly into each zucchini boat. Drizzle some olive oil and sprinkle a little salt over the top. Put in the oven and bake for 25–30 minutes or until the mixture is golden on top.

6. Serve with a fresh mixed salad and enjoy while warm.

Tip: *if there is any turkey mixture left, store it in the fridge. You can serve the leftovers on top of toasted Rice Flour Bread with Chia & Flaxseed (see page 229).*

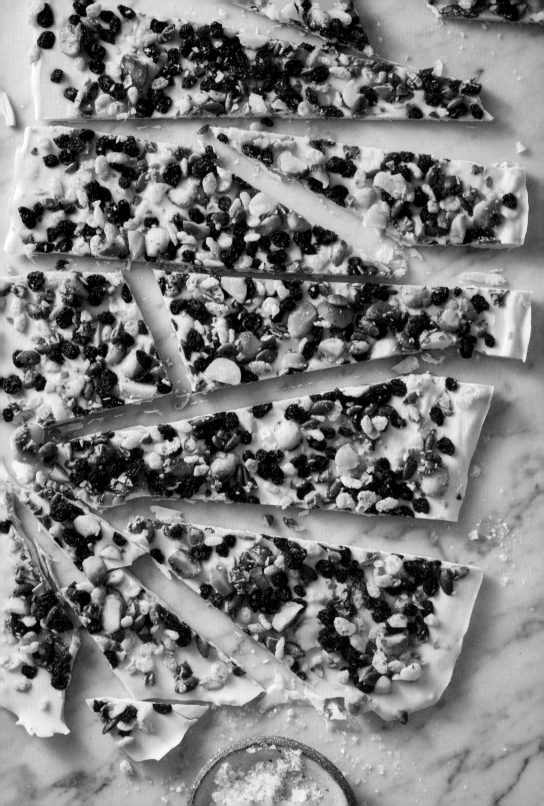

White chocolate bark
with blackcurrants & macadamia

Serves 6   gf   wf   df   sf   vt

1 tbsp coconut oil

½ cup macadamias

¼ cup pumpkin seeds

2 large white chocolate blocks

½ cup dried blackcurrants

¼ cup puffed rice cereal

Pinch of sea salt

1. Heat the coconut oil in a small pan over medium–high heat. Toast the macadamias and pumpkin seeds until golden, about 4–5 minutes. Set aside to cool completely. Once cooled, roughly chop the nut mixture.

2. Bring a pot of water to the boil and add a bowl on top. Add the white chocolate and melt, stirring frequently with a spatula.

3. Pour the melted chocolate onto a small, lined baking tray. Scatter over the nut mixture, blackcurrants, puffed rice and sea salt, then place in the fridge to set.

4. When set, roughly chop it or break it up into desired pieces. This keeps for two weeks in the fridge – if it lasts that long!

Rosemary potato crisps

Serves 4   gf   wf   df   sf   vt   ve

4 russet potatoes, very thinly sliced
  (use a mandolin)

3 tbsp extra-virgin olive oil

3 tbsp fresh or dried rosemary,
  finely chopped

1 tsp garlic powder

4 tbsp sea salt

1. Preheat the oven to 220°C (425°F).

2. In a large mixing bowl, toss the potatoes in the olive oil, rosemary, garlic powder and salt.

3. Transfer the mixture to a lined baking tray and evenly spread across, making sure the potatoes don't overlap. Put the tray in the oven and bake until the potatoes are crisp and golden, about 25–30 minutes, turning the potatoes over halfway.

4. Remove from oven and let cool completely. Enjoy as a healthy afternoon snack!

Snacks

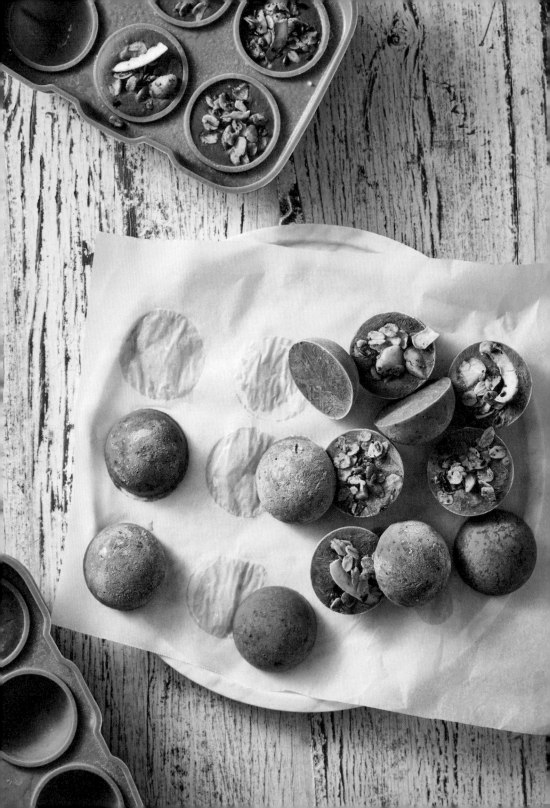

Roasted spiced macadamias & pecans

Makes 4 cups   gf   wf   df   sf   vt   ve

2 cups macadamias

2 cups pecans

2 tbsp macadamia or extra-virgin
   olive oil

1 tbsp curry powder

1 tsp ground cumin

1 tsp ground sweet paprika

1 tsp ground turmeric

1 tbsp salt

1. Preheat the oven to 180°C (350°F).

2. Put the nuts in a mixing bowl then season with the oil, spices and salt, tossing well.

3. Spread out the nuts on a lined baking tray. Bake for 25–30 minutes or until
    lightly golden, shaking the tray occasionally.

4. Remove tray from oven and separate the nuts using a wooden spoon. Set aside
    and let cool.

5. Store in an airtight jar or container. Enjoy any time!

Snacks

Blueberry & basil smoothie bites

Makes 24 bites   gf   wf   df   sf   vt   ve

1 cup frozen blueberries

1 cup frozen dragon fruit (pitaya)
   chunks

1 cup coconut milk

2 tbsp coconut yoghurt

2 tbsp Love Your Gut powder[1]

1 tbsp chia seeds

6 basil leaves

Pinch of sea salt

Coconut oil spray

Maple Macadamia Granola (see
   page 187), for topping (optional)

1. Put all the ingredients in a blender and blend on high until smooth and creamy.

2. Lightly spray a 24-semi sphere silicone mould with coconut oil and pour mixture
    in. If you wish, you could top the smoothie bites with granola if using. Place
    in the freezer until frozen, about 1–2 hours. Keep frozen until ready to grab as
    a delicious snack!

[1]superchargeyourgut.com

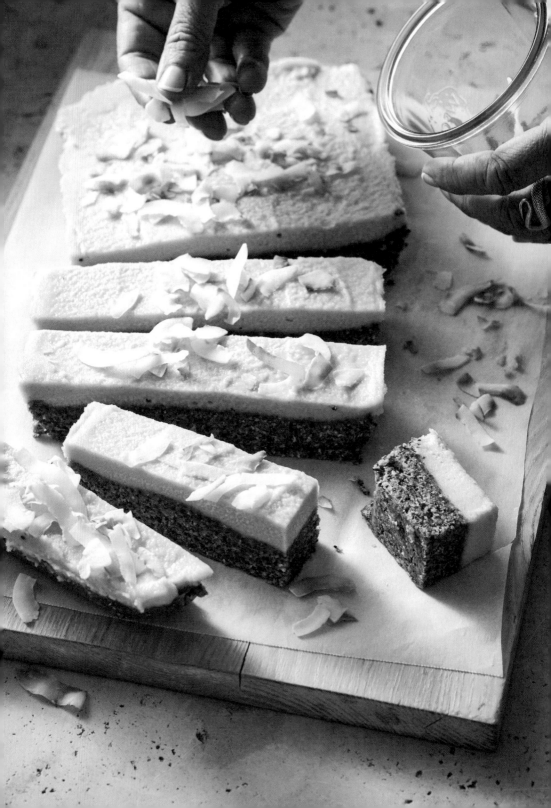

Coconut, cranberry & macadamia slice

Makes 12   gf wf df sf vt ve

BASE

1½ cups dried cranberries, plus
  extra to garnish

1 cup roasted macadamias, plus
  extra to garnish

½ cup chia seeds

1 cup raw pecans

½ cup hemp seeds

½ cup rolled oats

½ cup desiccated coconut, plus
  extra to garnish

1 tsp cinnamon

1 tsp sea salt

½ cup liquid coconut oil

2 tbsp maple syrup

TOPPING

1½ cups macadamias

⅔ cup organic full-fat coconut
  cream

2 tbsp maple syrup

1. Line a shallow baking tray with baking paper.
2. To make the base, put all the dry ingredients in a food processor and blitz until it forms a crumbly texture. Add the coconut oil and maple syrup and blitz to combine, scraping down the sides of the processor with a spatula as necessary.
3. Scoop the mixture onto the lined baking tray and place in the freezer for 30 minutes.
4. Meanwhile, make the topping by combining all the ingredients into a food processor and blend until smooth.
5. When firm, remove the base from the freezer and add the topping, using the back of a spoon to smooth the top. Sprinkle extra cranberries, macadamias and desiccated coconut on top to garnish. Return the slice to the fridge for 30 minutes or until set.
6. Cut into slices and serve. Keep in an airtight container in the fridge for up to 1 week, or 2 weeks in the freezer.

Snacks

Ricotta rice cakes with passionfruit & honey

Serves 1   gf wf df sf vt

2 tbsp ricotta

1 tbsp chia seeds

2 tbsp honey

1 tbsp water

½ tsp sea salt

2 brown rice cakes

2 tbsp passionfruit pulp

1 tsp shredded coconut

3 fresh mint leaves, torn

1. Combine the ricotta, chia seeds, 1 tbsp honey, water and salt in a mixing bowl. Whisk thoroughly until the ricotta is smooth.

2. Spread the ricotta mixture onto each rice cake. Spoon passionfruit pulp over each rice cake. Sprinkle coconut and drizzle the remaining honey on top. Serve with torn mint leaves scattered over.

Air-fryer zucchini fries

Serves 4   gf   wf   df   sf   vt   ve

2 medium zucchini, sliced lengthwise into sticks

Sea salt

½ cup flaxseed
(linseed) meal

1 tbsp cumin ground

1 tbsp onion powder

Olive oil spray

1. Preheat an air fryer to 200°C (400°F).

2. Place the zucchini sticks on a large plate and season heavily with salt. Let sit for
   5 minutes. (This will help the flaxseed meal to stick.)

3. Combine the flaxseed meal, cumin, onion powder and 1 tbsp sea salt in
   a shallow bowl. Dredge the zucchini sticks in the flaxseed mixture one at a time,
   then place the sticks in the air-fryer basket. Make sure they are laying separately;
   you can cook them in batches if you need.

4. Spray the sticks generously with olive oil. Cook for 8 minutes or until golden.
   Repeat with the remaining zucchini sticks. Serve immediately.

Snacks

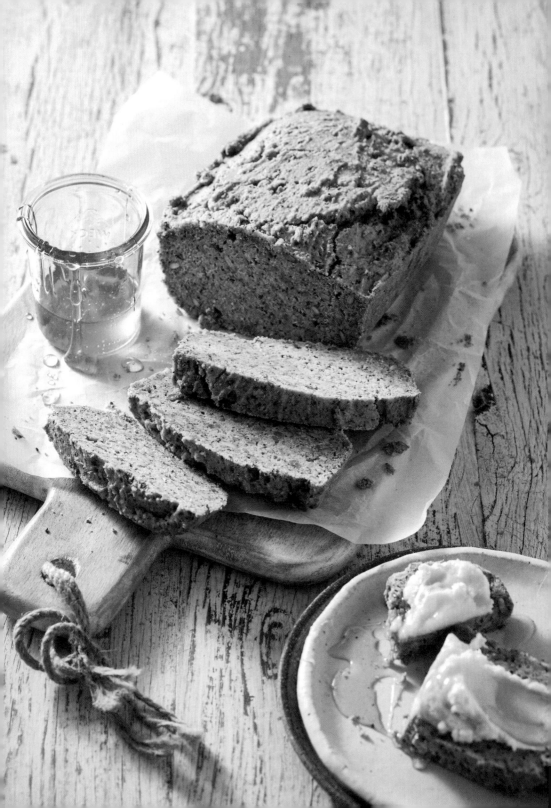

Rice flour bread with chia & flaxseed

Makes 1 loaf   gf wf df sf vt

2⅓ cups rice flour

¾ cup mixed sunflower seeds and pumpkin seeds

¼ cup flaxseed (linseed) meal

¼ cup chia seeds

1½ tsp baking powder

½ tsp sea salt

4 eggs

½ cup filtered water

⅓ cup coconut milk

4 tbsp unsalted butter, melted

1 tbsp maple syrup

1 tsp apple cider vinegar

1. Preheat the oven to 175°C (345°F). Grease and flour a 20 x 9 cm (8 x 3½ inch) loaf tin.

2. Combine the rice flour, seeds, flaxseed meal, baking powder and salt in a bowl and mix until combined.

3. In a separate large bowl, use an electric mixer to beat the eggs for about 2 minutes until pale and fluffy. Stir in the water, coconut milk, melted butter, maple syrup and apple cider vinegar. Pour the wet ingredients into the dry ingredients and stir well to combine.

4. Spoon the mixture into the prepared loaf tin. Bake in the oven for 40 minutes or until a skewer inserted in the centre of the loaf comes out clean.

5. Turn out onto a wire rack to cool. This loaf will keep for 1 week in the fridge or 2 months in the freezer.

Other

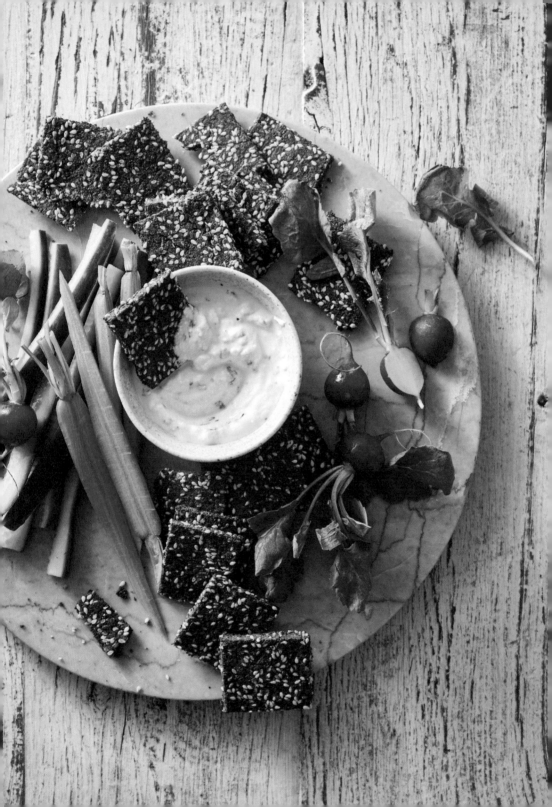

Ginger, turmeric & sesame crackers

Makes 35   gf wf df sf vt

1¼ cups flaxseed (linseed) meal

½ cup sesame seeds

1 tsp grated fresh ginger or ½ tsp ground ginger

1 tsp ground turmeric

½ tsp sea salt

1 egg

1½ tbsp extra-virgin olive oil

1. Preheat the oven to 175°C (345°F). Grease a baking tray.
2. Combine the flaxseed meal, sesame seeds, ginger, turmeric and salt in a large bowl.
3. In a small bowl, whisk the egg then slowly add the olive oil in a thin stream while still whisking. Pour the egg mixture into the dry ingredients and mix to form a firm dough. If it is too dry to roll out, add a little filtered water.
4. Roll out the dough on a sheet of baking paper to a thin rectangle about 25 x 35 cm (10 x 14 inches). Place the prepared baking tray face down over the dough then invert both together so the dough is in the middle of the tray and the paper is on top. Peel off the baking paper and cut the dough into 5 cm (2 inch) squares using a sharp knife.
5. Bake for 15–20 minutes until crisp and golden. Allow to cool completely before eating.

Tip: *I usually store these crackers in an airtight container for 3–4 days, but they also do well in the fridge and last up to 2 weeks. Check and see if you have any reactions after eating eggs. If you're okay with including eggs in your low-histamine diet, then these crackers are a delicious addition.*

Other

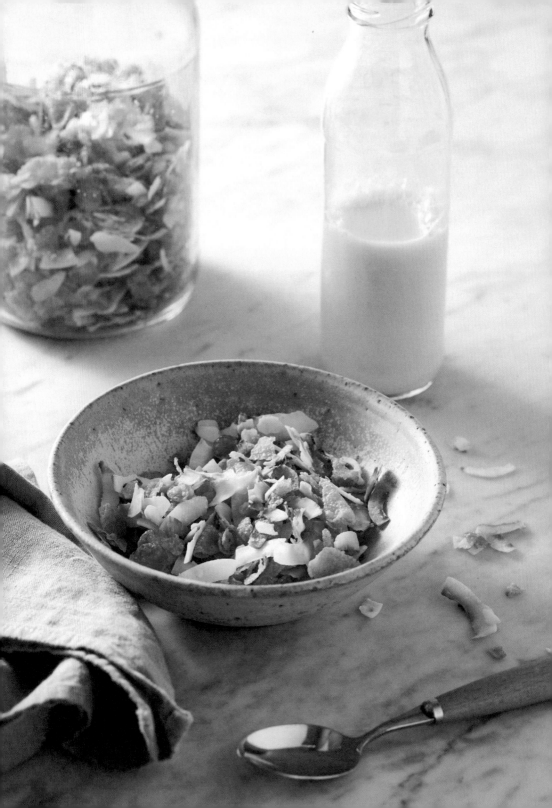

Low-histamine food list

Note: use all ingredients with an * in small amounts to begin with. Check for any reactions and if you can tolerate them.

acerola

agave syrup

*almond

amaranth

anise, aniseed

apple

*apple cider vinegar

apricot

artichoke

arugula (rocket)

asparagus

*bamboo shoots

*barley

basil

beef (fresh)

beetroot (fresh)

black caraway

blackberry

blackcurrants

blueberries

bok choi

*boysenberry

brazil nuts

broccoli

*brussels sprouts

butter

cabbage (green or white)

capsicum (red, yellow, orange, green)

caraway

cardamom

carrot

*cashews

cassava

cassava flour

cauliflower

celery

celery cabbage

chamomile tea

*cheese (soft cheeses)

cherries

chestnut

chestnut, sweet

chia seed

chicken (organic, fresh)

chicory

*chives

chocolate (white only)

*cinnamon

cloves

*cocoa butter

coconut meat

coconut milk

coconut oil

coriander

corn

cornflakes

cranberries

cranberry nectar

cream (sweet, without additives)

*cream cheeses (plain, without additives)

*cress

*cucumber

*curry

*dates (dried, desiccated)

*dill

dragon fruit (pitaya)

duck (organic, freshly cooked)

*egg white

*egg yolk

elderflower cordial

endive

fennel

fennel flower (*Nigella sativa*)

*feta cheese

*figs (fresh or dried)

fish (fresh)

233

flaxseed (linseed)
fructose
garlic
ginger
glucose
goat's milk
gooseberries
*gouda cheese
gourds
grapes
*green beans
*green peas
*green split peas
*green tea
*hazelnuts
hemp seeds
*herbal teas with
  medicinal herbs
  (check ingredients)
honey
*horseradish
juniper berries
kale
Kamut
*kohlrabi
lamb (organic,
  freshly cooked)
lamb's lettuce,
  corn salad
*leeks
lettuce (iceberg)
lettuce (head and
  leaf lettuces)
lime flower

lychees
macadamias
*mangoes
maple syrup
marrow
*mascarpone cheese
*mate tea
melon (rock,
  honeydew)
*milk (lactose-free,
  pasteurised, UHT)
millet
minced meat (fresh)
mineral water, still
mint
morello cherries
*mozzarella cheese
*mulberries
*mung beans
  (germinated,
  sprouting)
*mushrooms
  (different types)
napa cabbage
*nashi pears
*nectarines
Nigella sativa
  (oil, seed)
*nutmeg
*oat drink, oat milk
oats
olive oil (extra-virgin)
*olives
onions

oregano
ostrich meat
pak choi
palm kernel oil
palm sugar
paprika (sweet)
parsley
parsnips
passionfruit
*pasta
*pawpaw
pea shoots
peaches
pearl sago
*pears
pecans
peppermint tea
Persian cumin
persimmons
*pine nuts
*pistachios
*plums
pomegranates
poppy seeds
pork (fresh)
potatoes
poultry meat
*prickly pear
*prunes
psyllium seed husks
puffed rice cereal
pumpkin seed oil
pumpkin seeds

pumpkins
  (various varieties)
quail
quark
quinces
*quinine
quinoa
radish (red,
  round, white)
raisins (no sulphur)
raspberries (contain
  histamine but also
  contain quercetin,
  an antihistamine)
raw milk
redcurrants, currants
rice

rice cakes
*rice milk, rice drink

rice noodles
ricotta cheese
Roman coriander
Roman coriander oil
rooibos tea
*Roquefort cheese
*rosehips
rosemary
*rye
safflower oil
sage
sago
*Savoy cabbage
*sesame
sheep's milk
*snow peas
*soda water
*soft cheese
sour cherries
*sour cream

spelt
squashes
*star anise
starch
stevia
*stinging nettle
  herbal tea
sweet potatoes
sweetcorn
thyme
tiger nuts
*trout
turkey
turmeric
*turnips
*vanilla beans
  (extract)
veal (fresh)
*venison
zucchini

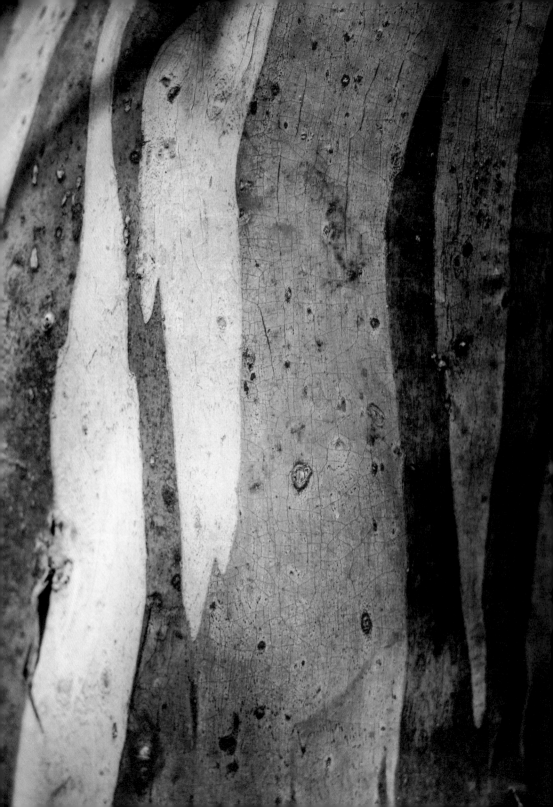

Glossary

ACE2 RECEPTORS: proteins on the cell surface that SARS-CoV-2 uses to enter and infect human cells

ACUTE: refers to a condition or illness that develops suddenly and has a short duration

ADAPTIVE IMMUNITY: the body's ability to recognise and defend against specific pathogens, often through producing antibodies

ANTI-INFLAMMATORIES: medications or substances that reduce inflammation

ANTIBODIES: proteins produced by the immune system to neutralise or target foreign substances, such as viruses or bacteria

ANTIGENS: molecules that trigger an immune response and are typically found on the surface of pathogens

ANTIHISTAMINES: medications that counteract the effects of histamine

ANTIOXIDANT: compounds that help to protect cells from damage caused by oxidative stress and free radicals

ATHEROSCLEROSIS: build-up of plaque in the arteries, leading to reduced blood flow

AUTOANTIBODIES: antibodies that mistakenly target and attack the body's own tissues; often seen in autoimmune diseases

AUTOIMMUNE DISEASE: condition in which the immune system mistakenly attacks the body's own tissues

AUTONOMIC NERVOUS SYSTEM: the part of the nervous system that controls involuntary functions, such as heart rate. Dysfunction occurs when the regulation of these functions is abnormal

AUTOPHAGY: cellular process that removes damaged or dysfunctional components to maintain cell health

B CELL: type of white blood cell responsible for producing antibodies

CARDIOVASCULAR SYSTEM: body system responsible for circulating blood, including the heart and blood vessels

CHEMOKINES: signalling proteins that play a role in immune cell migration

CHRONIC: refers to a long-lasting, often persistent condition or disease

CIRCADIAN RHYTHM: the body's natural, 24-hour biological clock that regulates sleep–wake cycles and other physiological processes

COGNITIVE DYSFUNCTION: impairment in brain functions, such as memory and thinking

CORTISOL: hormone produced by the adrenal glands that plays a role in stress response and metabolism

COVID-19: disease caused by the SARS-CoV-2 virus, characterised by respiratory and systemic symptoms

CRANIAL POLYNEURITIS: inflammation of multiple cranial nerves, leading to various neurological symptoms

CROSS REACTIVITY: when the immune system responds to a substance similar to the intended target

CYTOKINES: Signalling molecules involved in the immune response. A cytokine storm is an excessive and harmful release of cytokines

DORMANT VIRUSES: Viruses that are in a state of latency within the host, not actively replicating

DOWNREGULATION: process of decreasing the activity or expression of a gene or receptor

DYSAUTONOMIA: dysfunction of the autonomic nervous system, leading to problems with regulating bodily functions

EMBOLISM: A blockage in a blood vessel, typically caused by a blood clot or other foreign material

ENDOTHELIUM: the inner lining of blood vessels, essential for vascular health

FATIGUE: persistent feeling of tiredness or exhaustion

FLAVONOIDS: group of natural compounds with antioxidant properties, found in many plants

GASTROINTESTINAL SYSTEM: system responsible for digestion and nutrient absorption

GENE EXPRESSION: process by which genetic information is used to create proteins

GENETIC PREDISPOSITION: an individual's genetic susceptibility to a certain condition

GERD: gastro-oesophageal reflux disease, a condition in which stomach acid flows back into the oesophagus

GUILLAIN-BARRÉ SYNDROME: rare neurological disorder that leads to muscle weakness and paralysis

GUT DYSBIOSIS: imbalance in the microbial community in the digestive system

HISTAMINE: chemical involved in allergic reactions

HYPERCOAGULABILITY: a state of increased blood clotting

HYPERTENSION: high blood pressure, a risk factor for cardiovascular diseases

HYPOXEMIA: low oxygen levels in the blood

HYPOXIA: deficiency of oxygen in body tissues

IMMUNE CELL MIGRATION: movement of immune cells to the site of an infection or inflammation

IMMUNE SYSTEM: the body's defence system against pathogens and foreign substances

INFLAMMATION: the body's response to infection or injury. Hyperinflammation is an excessive inflammatory response

LEAKY GUT SYNDROME: condition in which the lining of the gut becomes more permeable than normal

MAST CELLS: immune cells that play a role in allergic reactions

METABOLISM: set of chemical reactions that occur within an organism to maintain life

MICROBIOTA: community of microorganisms living in a specific environment (called a microbiome) such as the gut

MICROCLOT: A small blood clot, potentially contributing to thrombotic (blood-clotting) events

MITOCHONDRIA: organelles within cells that produce energy

MUSCULOSKELETAL SYSTEM: body system that includes muscles and bones

MYOCARDITIS: inflammation of the heart muscle

NATURAL KILLER CELLS: immune cells that can kill infected or cancerous cells

NEURO-OPHTHALMOLOGICAL DISORDER: disorder affecting both the nervous system and eyes

NEUROINFLAMMATION: inflammation in the nervous system, often associated with neurological disorders

NEUROLOGICAL SYSTEM: body system that controls the nervous system, including the brain and spinal cord

NEUROMUSCULAR JUNCTION DISORDER: condition affecting the connection between nerves and muscles

NEUROSENSORY HEARING LOSS: loss of hearing related to nerve or sensory issues

OLFACTORY: relating to the sense of smell

OPPORTUNISTIC: referring to pathogens that take advantage of weakened immune systems

ORTHOSTATIC INTOLERANCE: condition in which a person has difficulty standing upright due to changes in blood pressure

OXIDATIVE STRESS: imbalance between free radicals and antioxidants, leading to cellular damage

PALPITATIONS: sensations of rapid, irregular or pounding heartbeats

PARASYMPATHETIC NERVOUS SYSTEM: part of the autonomic nervous system responsible for rest and relaxation

PATHOGENS: microorganisms or agents that cause disease

PERICARDITIS: inflammation of the lining around the heart

PERIPHERAL NEUROPATHY: damage to nerves outside of the brain and spinal cord (the central nervous system)

PERMEABILITY: ability of a membrane or barrier to allow substances to pass through

PNEUMONIA: inflammation of the lungs, often caused by infection

POLYPHENOLS: group of natural compounds found in plants with potential health benefits

POST-VIRAL FATIGUE SYNDROME: symptoms such as fatigue persisting after a viral infection

POSTURAL TACHYCARDIA SYNDROME: condition characterised by an excessive increase in heart rate upon standing

PREBIOTICS: compounds that promote the growth of beneficial gut bacteria

PROBIOTICS: live microorganisms that live in the gut and provide health benefits

PROTEASE: enzymes that break down proteins

PSYCHOLOGY: study of the mind and human behaviour, often related to the emotional and mental aspects of health

PULMONARY FIBROSIS: scarring of lung tissue, which can affect lung function

RESPIRATORY SYSTEM: body system responsible for breathing

SARS-CoV-2: virus responsible for COVID-19

SMALL FIBRE NEUROPATHY: damage to small nerve fibres that can lead to various sensory symptoms

SPIKE PROTEIN: protein on the surface of SARS-CoV-2 that it uses to enter human cells

SYMPATHETIC NERVOUS SYSTEM: part of the autonomic nervous system responsible for the fight-or-flight response

SYNBIOTIC: a combination of prebiotics and probiotics, working together to improve gut health

T CELL: type of white blood cell important for immune response

TACHYCARDIA: abnormally rapid heart rate

THROMBOTIC: related to the formation of blood clots

TRYPTASE: enzyme released during allergic reactions and in mast cell disorders

VAGUS NERVE: cranial nerve that plays a key role in regulating various bodily functions

VESTIBULAR REHABILITATION: therapy to treat balance and dizziness issues

VIRAL LOAD: amount of virus present in the body, often used to measure disease progression or transmission

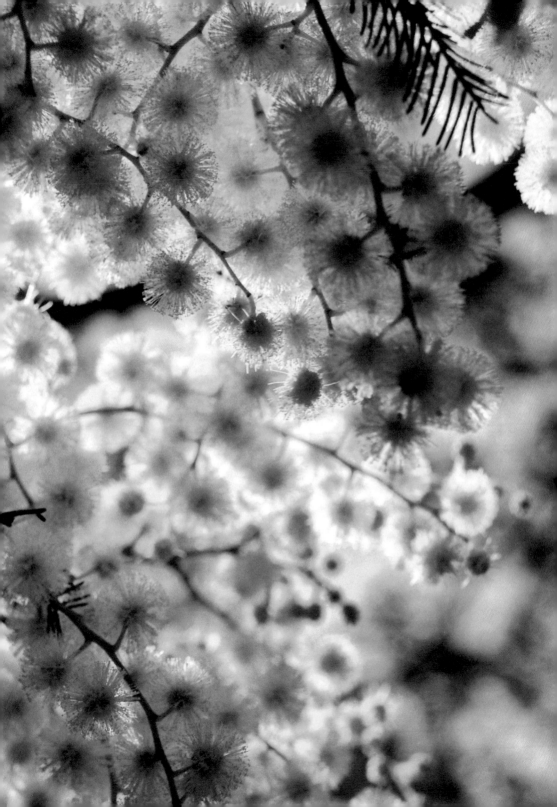

Endnotes

1. Marcin Sekowski, Małgorzata Gambin, Karolina Hansen, et al. 'Risk of developing post-traumatic stress disorder in severe COVID-19 survivors, their families and frontline healthcare workers: what should mental health specialists prepare for?' *Frontiers in Psychiatry*, 2021, vol. 12, art. 562899. https://www.frontiersin.org/articles/10.3389/fpsyt.2021.562899/full

2. Brunilda Nazario, 'Coronavirus and COVID-19: what you should know', *WebMD*, 26 December 2022, https://www.webmd.com/covid/news/20211118/millions-worldwide-long-covid-study

3. Elisa Perego, 'Two years ago today the term #LongCovid was first used as a Twitter hashtag.' Twitter/X post, 21 May 2022. https://twitter.com/elisaperego78/status/1527740626934063104?lang=en

4. World Health Organization (WHO), 'Coronavirus disease (COVID-19): post COVID-19 condition', WHO website, 28 March 2023. https://www.who.int/news-room/questions-and-answers/item/coronavirus-disease-(covid-19)-post-covid-19-condition

5. Hannah E. Davis, Gina S. Assaf, Lisa McCorkell, et al. 'Characterizing long COVID in an international cohort: 7 months of symptoms and their impact', *eClinicalMedicine*, 2021, vol. 38, art. 101019. https://www.thelancet.com/journals/eclinm/article/PIIS2589-5370(21)00299-6/fulltext

6. J. De la Cruz-Enríquez, E. Rojas-Morales, M. G. Ruíz-García, et al. 'SARS-CoV-2 induces mitochondrial dysfunction and cell death by oxidative stress/inflammation in leukocytes of COVID-19 patients', *Free Radical Research*, 2021, vol. 55, no. 9–10, pp. 982–995. https://www.tandfonline.com/doi/abs/10.1080/10715762.2021.2005247

7. H. E. Davis, L. McCorkell, J. M. Vogel, et al. 'Long COVID: major findings, mechanisms and recommendations', *Nature Reviews Microbiology*, 2023, vol. 21, no. 3, pp. 133–146. https://www.nature.com/articles/s41579-022-00846-2

8. Hannah E. Davis, Lisa McCorkell, Julia M. Vogel, et al. 'Long COVID: major findings, mechanisms and recommendations', *Nature Reviews: Microbiology*, 2023, vol. 21, no. 3, pp. 133–146. https://www.ncbi.nlm.nih.gov/pmc/articles/PMC9839201/

9. Stephani Sutherland, 'Long COVID now looks like a neurological disease, helping doctors to focus treatments', *Scientific American*, 1 March 2023. https://www.scientificamerican.com/article/long-covid-now-looks-like-a-neurological-disease-helping-doctors-to-focus-treatments

10. Lars Ittner and Yazi Ke, 'COVID-19 could cause long-term neuron damage: new study', *The Lighthouse*, 8 June 2023. https://lighthouse.mq.edu.au/article/june-2023/covid-19-could-cause-long-term-neuron-damage-new-study

11. Lars Ittner and Yazi Ke, 'COVID-19 could cause long-term neuron damage: new study,' Th*e Lighthouse*, 8 June 2023. https://lighthouse.mq.edu.au/article/june-2023/covid-19-could-cause-long-term-neuron-damage-new-study

12. Malavika Lingeswaran, Taru Goyal, Raghumoy Ghosh, et al. 'Inflammation, immunity and immunogenetics in COVID-19: a narrative review', *Indian Journal of Clinical Biochemistry*, 2020, vol. 35, no. 3, pp. 260–273. https://www.ncbi.nlm.nih.gov/pmc/articles/PMC7275846/

13. Denise Goh, Jeffrey C. T. Lim, Sonia B. Fernaíndez, et al. 'Case report: persistence of residual antigen and RNA of the SARS-CoV-2 virus in tissues of two patients with long COVID', *Frontiers in Immunology*, 2022, vol. 13. https://www.frontiersin.org/articles/10.3389/fimmu.2022.939989/

14. Umberto Maccio, Annelies S. Zinkernagel, Reto Schuepbach, et al. 'Long-term persisting SARS-CoV-2 RNA and pathological findings: lessons learnt from a series of 35 COVID-19 autopsies', *Frontiers in Medicine*, 2022, vol. 9, art. 778489. https://www.ncbi.nlm.nih.gov/pmc/articles/PMC8865372/

15. Hannah E. Davis, Gina S. Assaf, Lisa McCorkell, et al. 'Characterizing long COVID in an international cohort: 7 months of symptoms and their impact', *eClinicalMedicine*, 2021, vol. 38, art. 101019. https://www.thelancet.com/journals/eclinm/article/PIIS2589-5370(21)00299-6/fulltext

16. Nina Lichtenberg, 'NIH study identifies features of Long COVID neurological symptoms', *National Institutes of Neurological Disorders and Stroke*, 5 May 2023. https://www.nih.gov/news-events/news-releases/nih-study-identifies-features-long-covid-neurological-symptoms

17. Brad Ryan, 'Long COVID research pledge prompts push to consider mystery links to other illness', *ABC News*, 25 April 2023. https://www.abc.net.au/news/2023-04-25/long-covid-report-sparks-push-for-research-into-linked-illnesses/102262582

18. Rafael Cardoso Maciel Costa Silva, Jhones Sousa Ribeiro, Gustavo Peixoto Duarte da Silva, et al. 'Autophagy modulators in coronavirus diseases: a double strike in viral burden and inflammation', *Frontiers in Cellular and Infection Microbiology*, 2022, vol. 12, art. 845368. https://www.frontiersin.org/articles/10.3389/fcimb.2022.845368/full

19. Sharon Reynolds, 'Immune response found in many with COVID-19', *National Institutes of Health*, 28 September 2021. https://www.nih.gov/news-events/nih-research-matters/autoimmune-response-found-many-covid-19

20. Vasiliki Tsampasian, Hussein Elghazaly, Rahul Chattopadhyay, et al. 'Risk factors associated with post–COVID-19 condition: a systematic review and meta-analysis', *JAMA Internal Medicine*, 2023, vol. 183, no. 6, pp. 566–580. https://jamanetwork.com/journals/jamainternalmedicine/fullarticle/2802877

21. Brad Ryan, 'Long COVID research pledge prompts push to consider mystery links to other illness', *ABC News*, 25 April 2023. https://www.abc.net.au/news/2023-04-25/long-covid-report-sparks-push-for-research-into-linked-illnesses/102262582

22. Sivananthan Manoharan and Lee Ying Ying, 'Epstein Barr virus reactivation during COVID-19 hospitalization significantly increased mortality/death in SARS-CoV-2(+)/EBV(+) than SARS-CoV-2(+)/EBV(−) patients: a comparative meta-analysis', *International Journal of Clinical Practice*, 2023, art. 1068000. https://www.ncbi.nlm.nih.gov/pmc/articles/PMC9904914/

23. Aristo Vojdani, Elroy Vojdani, Evan Saidara, et al. 'Persistent SARS-CoV-2 infection, EBV, HHV-6 and other factors may contribute to inflammation and autoimmunity in long COVID. *Viruses*, 2023, vol.15, no. 2, p. 400. https://www.ncbi.nlm.nih.gov/pmc/articles/PMC9967513/

24. Matthew P. Giannetti, Emily Weller, Iván Alvarez-Twose, et al. 'COVID-19 infection in patients with mast cell disorders including mastocytosis does not impact mast cell activation symptoms', *Journal of Allergy and Clinical Immunology: In Practice*, 2021, vol. 9, no. 5, pp. 2083–2086.

25. Yun-Ju Lai, Shou-Hou Liu, Sumatchara Manachevakul, et al. 'Biomarkers in long COVID-19: a systematic review', *Frontiers in Medicine*, 2023, vol. 10, art. 1085988. https://www.frontiersin.org/articles/10.3389/fmed.2023.1085988/full

26. Sindhu Mohandas, Prasanna Jagannathan, Timothy J. Henrich, et al. 'Immune mechanisms underlying COVID-19 pathology and post-acute sequelae of SARS-CoV-2 infection (PASC)', *eLife*, 2023, vol. 12, art. e86014. https://elifesciences.org/articles/86014.pdf

27. L. B. Afrin, L. B. Weinstock and G. J. Molderings, 'Covid-19 hyperinflammation and post-Covid-19 illness may be rooted in mast cell activation syndrome', *International Journal of Infectious Diseases*, 2020, vol. 100, pp. 327–332. https://pubmed.ncbi.nlm.nih.gov/32920235/

28. M. P. Giannetti, E. Weller, I. Alvarez-Twose, et al, 'COVID-19 infection in patients with mast cell disorders including mastocytosis does not impact mast cell activation symptoms', *The Journal of Allergy and Clinical Immunology*. In Practice, 2021, vol. 9, no. 5, pp. 2083–2086. https://www.ncbi.nlm.nih.gov/pmc/articles/PMC7899934/

29. Yun-Ju Lai, Shou-Hou Liu, Sumatchara Manachevakul, et al. 'Biomarkers in long COVID-19: a systematic review', *Frontiers in Medicine*, 2023, vol. 10, art. 1085988. https://www.frontiersin.org/articles/10.3389/fmed.2023.1085988/full

30. S. W. Xu, I. Ilyas and J.-P. Weng, 'Endothelial dysfunction in COVID-19: an overview of evidence, biomarkers, mechanisms and potential therapies', *Acta Pharmacologica Sinica*, 2023, vol. 44, pp. 695–709. https://www.nature.com/articles/s41401-022-00998-0

31. S. Montazersaheb, S. M. Hosseiniyan Khatibi, M. S. Hejazi, et al. 'COVID-19 infection: an overview on cytokine storm and related interventions', *Virology Journal*, 2022, vol. 19, p. 92. https://virologyj.biomedcentral.com/articles/10.1186/s12985-022-01814-1

32. M. Madjid, P. Safavi-Naeini, S. D. Solomon, et al. 'Potential effects of coronaviruses on the cardiovascular system: a review', *JAMA Cardiology*, 2020, vol. 5, no. 7, | pp. 831–840. https://jamanetwork.com/journals/jamacardiology/fullarticle/2763846

33. K. O. Mohammad, A. Lin, and J. B. C. Rodriguez, 'Cardiac manifestations of post-acute COVID-19 infection', *Current Cardiology Reports*, 2022, vol. 24, no. 12, pp. 1775–1783. https://www.ncbi.nlm.nih.gov/pmc/articles/PMC9628458/

34. L. Townsend, H. Fogarty, A. Dyer, et al. 'Prolonged elevation of D-dimer levels in convalescent COVID-19 patients is independent of the acute phase response,' *Journal of Thromosis and Haemostasis*, 2021, vol. 19, pp. 1064–1070. https://pubmed.ncbi.nlm.nih.gov/33587810/

35. Sasan Andalib, José Biller, Mario Di Napoli, et al. 'Peripheral nervous system manifestations associated with COVID-19', *Current Neurology and Neuroscience Reports*, 2021, vol. 21, no. 3, art. 9. https://www.ncbi.nlm.nih.gov/pmc/articles/PMC7882462/

36. L. M. Grobbelaar, C. Venter, M. Vlok, et al. 'SARS-CoV-2 spike protein S1 induces fibrin(ogen) resistant to fibrinolysis: implications for microclot formation in COVID-19', *Bioscience Reports*, 2021, vol. 41, no. 8, art. PMC8380922. https://www.ncbi.nlm.nih.gov/pmc/articles/PMC8380922/

37. M. Dani, A. Dirksen, P. Taraborrelli, et al. 'Autonomic dysfunction in "long COVID": rationale, physiology and management strategies', *Clinical Medicine (London, England)*, 2021, vol. 21, no. 1, pp. e63–e67. https://www.ncbi.nlm.nih.gov/pmc/articles/PMC7850225/

38. Ted Bosworth, 'Explanation proposed for long-COVID symptoms in the CNS', *MD Edge/Neurology*, 24 April 2023. https://www.mdedge.com/neurology/article/262566/long-covid/explanation-proposed-long-covid-symptoms-cns

39. S. R. Stein, S. C. Ramelli, A. Grazioli, et al. 'SARS-CoV-2 infection and persistence in the human body and brain at autopsy', *Nature*, 2022, vol. 612, pp. 758–763. https://www.nature.com/articles/s41586-022-05542-y

40. Mariane Daou, Hussein Kannout, Mariam Khalili, et al. 'Analysis of SARS-CoV-2 viral loads in stool samples and nasopharyngeal swabs from COVID-19 patients in the United Arab Emirates', *PLoS One*, 2022, vol. 17, no. 9, art. e0274961. https://www.ncbi.nlm.nih.gov/pmc/articles/PMC9499247/

41. B. Raman, D. A. Bluemke, T. F. Lüscher, et al. 'Long COVID: post-acute sequelae of COVID-19 with a cardiovascular focus', *European Heart Journal*, 2022, vol. 43, no. 11, pp. 1157–1172. https://www.ncbi.nlm.nih.gov/pmc/articles/PMC8903393/

42. A. M. Eldokla, A. A. Mohamed-Hussein, A. M. Fouad, et al. 'Prevalence and patterns of symptoms of dysautonomia in patients with long-COVID syndrome: a cross-sectional study. *Annals of Clinical and Translational Neurology*, 2022, vol. 9, no. 6, pp. 778–785. https://www.ncbi.nlm.nih.gov/pmc/articles/PMC9110879/

43. Danielle Ellis, 'Study links long COVID to gut inflammation and serotonin deficiency', *News Medical: Life Sciences*, 16 October 2023. https://www.news-medical.net/news/20231016/Study-links-long-COVID-to-gut-inflammation-and-serotonin-deficiency.aspx

44. 'Make-up of gut microbiome may influence COVID-19 severity and immune response', *BMJ Newsroom*, 11 January 2021. https://www.bmj.com/company/newsroom/make-up-of-gut-microbiome-may-influence-covid-19-severity-and-immune-response/

45. Y. K. Yeoh, T. Zuo, G. C., Lui, et al. 'Gut microbiota composition reflects disease severity and dysfunctional immune responses in patients with COVID-19', *BMJ Gut*, 2021, vol. 70, pp. 698–706. https://gut.bmj.com/content/70/4/698

46. Cyndya Shibao, Carmen Arzubiaga, L. Jackson Roberts 2nd, et al. 'Hyperadrenergic postural tachycardia syndrome in mast cell activation disorders', *Hypertension*, 2005, vol. 45, no. 3, pp. 385–390. https://pubmed.ncbi.nlm.nih.gov/15710782/

47. Ikram Hussain, Gabriel Liu Yuan Cher, Muhammad Abbas Abid, et al. 'Role of gut microbiome in COVID-19: an insight into pathogenesis and therapeutic potential', *Frontiers in Immunology*, 2021, vol. 12, art. 765965. https://www.frontiersin.org/articles/10.3389/fimmu.2021.765965/full#B31

48. K. F. Budden, S. L. Gellatly, D. L. Wood, et al. 'Emerging pathogenic links between microbiota and the gut-lung axis', *Nature Reviews. Microbiology*, 2017, vol. 15, no. 1, pp. 55–63. https://pubmed.ncbi.nlm.nih.gov/27694885/

49. Donna M. Mancini, Danielle L. Brunjes, Anuradha Lala, et al. 'Use of cardiopulmonary stress testing for patients with unexplained dyspnea post–coronavirus disease', *JACC: Heart Failure*, 2021, vol. 9, no. 12, pp. 927–937. https://www.sciencedirect.com/science/article/pii/S2213177921004807

50. S. M. Khan, A. Shilen, K. M. Heslin, et al. 'SARS-CoV-2 infection and subsequent changes in the menstrual cycle among participants in the Arizona CoVHORT study', *American Journal of Obstetrics and Gynecology*, 2022, vol. 226, no. 2, pp. 270–273. https://pubmed.ncbi.nlm.nih.gov/34555320/

51. W. Wang, X. Su, Y. Ding, et al. 'Thyroid function abnormalities in COVID-19 patients', *Frontiers in Endocrinology*, 2021, vol. 11, art. 623792. https://www.ncbi.nlm.nih.gov/pmc/articles/PMC7933556/

52. R. Świątkowska-Stodulska, A. Berlińska and E. Puchalska-Reglińska, 'Cortisol as an independent predictor of unfavorable outcomes in hospitalized COVID-19 patients', *Biomedicines*, 2022, vol. 10, no. 7, p. 1527. https://www.ncbi.nlm.nih.gov/pmc/articles/PMC9313159/

53. L. Newson, R. Lewis and M. O'Hara, 'Long Covid and menopause – the important role of hormones in Long Covid must be considered', *Maturitas*, 2021, vol. 152, p. 74. https://www.ncbi.nlm.nih.gov/pmc/articles/PMC8522980/

54. M. Irwin, A. Mascovich, J. C. Gillin, et al. 'Partial sleep deprivation reduces natural killer cell activity in humans', *Psychosomatic Medicine*, 1994, vol. 56, no. 6, pp. 493–498. https://pubmed.ncbi.nlm.nih.gov/7871104/

55. K. Chandrasekhar, Jyoti Kapoor, and Sridhar Anishetty, 'A prospective, randomized double-blind, placebo-controlled study of safety and efficacy of a high-concentration full-spectrum extract of *Ashwagandha* root in reducing stress and anxiety in adults', 2012, vol. 34, no. 3, pp. 255–262. https://www.ncbi.nlm.nih.gov/pmc/articles/PMC3573577/

56. Benjamin Chen, Boris Julg, Sindhu Mohandras, et al. 'Viral persistence, reactivation, and mechanisms of long COVID', *eLife*, 2023, vol. 12, art. e86015. https://elifesciences.org/articles/86015

57. Joseph M. Grimes, Shaheer Khan, Mark Badeaux, et al. 'Arginine depletion as a therapeutic approach for patients with COVID-19', *International Journal of Infectious Diseases*, 2021, vol. 102, pp. 566–570. https://www.ncbi.nlm.nih.gov/pmc/articles/PMC7641537/

58. Francisca J. Allendes, Hugo S. Díaz, Fernando C. Ortiz, et al. 'Cardiovascular and autonomic dysfunction in long-COVID syndrome and the potential role of non-invasive therapeutic strategies on cardiovascular outcomes', *Frontiers in Medicine*, 2023, vol. 9, art. 1095249. https://www.frontiersin.org/articles/10.3389/fmed.2022.1095249/full

59. Kathleen Mikkelsen and Vasso Apostolopoulos, 'Vitamin B1, B2, B3, B5, and B6 and the immune system', in M. Mahmoudi and N. Rezaei (eds.) *Nutrition and Immunity*, Springer, 2019, pp.115–125. https://link.springer.com/chapter/10.1007/978-3-030-16073-9_7; Hira Sakoor, Jack Feehan, Kathleen Mikkelsen, et al. 'Be well: A potential role for vitamin B in COVID-19', *Maturitas*, 2020, vol. 144, pp.108–111. https://www.maturitas.org/article/S0378-5122(20)30348-0/fulltext

60. Thanutchaporn Kumrungsee, Peipei Zhang, Maesaya Chartkul, et al. 'Potential role of vitamin B6 in ameliorating the severity of COVID-19 and its complications', *Frontiers in Nutrition*, 2020, vol. 7, art. 562051. https://www.frontiersin.org/articles/10.3389/fnut.2020.562051/full

61. C. Vollbrach and K. Kraft, 'Feasibility of vitamin C in the treatment of post viral fatigue with focus on long COVID, based on a systematic review of IV vitamin C on fatigue', *Nutrients*, 2021, vol. 13, no. 4, p. 1154. https://www.ncbi.nlm.nih.gov/pmc/articles/PMC8066596/

62. Marlene Busko, 'Could vitamin D supplementation help in long COVID?' *Medscape*, 16 May 2023. https://www.medscape.com/viewarticle/992013

63. I. R. Hargreaves and D. Mantle, 'COVID-19, coenzyme Q10 and selenium', *Advances in Experimental Medicine and Biology*, 2021, vol. 1327, pp.161–168. https://pubmed.ncbi.nlm.nih.gov/34279837/

64. Sheila A. Doggrell, 'Lyprinol – is it a useful anti-inflammatory agent?', *Evidence-based Complementary and Alternative Medicine: eCAM*, 2011, vol. 2011, art. 307121. https://www.ncbi.nlm.nih.gov/pmc/articles/PMC3163099/

65. Adorata E. Coman, Alexandr Ceasovschih, Antoneta D. Petroaie, et al. 'The significance of low magnesium levels in COVID-19 patients', *Medicina*, 2022, vol. 59, no. 2, art. 279. https://www.mdpi.com/1648-9144/59/2/279

66. Zhongcheng Shi and Carolos A. Puyo, 'N-acetylcysteine to combat COVID-19: an evidence review', *Therapeutics and Clinical Risk Management*, 2020, vol. 16, pp. 1047–1055. https://www.ncbi.nlm.nih.gov/pmc/articles/PMC7649937/

67. Isabella Panfoli and Alfonson Esposito, 'Beneficial effect of polyphenols in COVID-19 and the ectopic F1FO-ATP synthase: is there a link?' *Journal of Cellular Biochemistry*, 2022, vol. 123, no. 8, pp. 1281–1284. https://onlinelibrary.wiley.com/doi/full/10.1002/jcb.30306

68. Amin Gasmi, Pavan K. Mujawdiya, Roman Lysiuk, et al. 'Quercetin in the prevention and treatment of coronavirus infections: a focus on SARS-CoV-2', *Pharmaceuticals (Basel, Switzerland)*, 2022, vol. 15, no. 9, art. 1049. https://www.ncbi.nlm.nih.gov/pmc/articles/PMC9504481/

69. Wolfgang J. Schnedl, Michael Schenk, Sonja Lackner, et al. 'Diamine oxidase supplementation improves symptoms in patients with histamine intolerance', *Food Science and Biotechnology*, 2019, vol. 28, no. 6, pp. 1779–1784. https://www.ncbi.nlm.nih.gov/pmc/articles/PMC6859183/

70. Hsin-Jung Wu and Eric Wu, 'The role of gut microbiota in immune homeostasis and autoimmunity', *Gut Microbes*, 2012, vol. 3, no. 1, pp. 4–14. https://www.ncbi.nlm.nih.gov/pmc/articles/PMC3337124/

71. Elden B. Thangam, Ebenezer A. Jemima, Himadri Singh, et al. 'The role of histamine and histamine receptors in mast cell-mediated allergy and inflammation: the hunt for new therapeutic targets', *Frontiers in Medicine*, 2018, vol. 9, art. 1873. https://www.frontiersin.org/articles/10.3389/fimmu.2018.01873/full

Acknowledgements

I would like to extend my heartfelt gratitude to the many individuals who have contributed to my latest exploration into the world of Long Covid. This endeavour has been a collaborative effort, and I am immensely thankful for the support and assistance I have received along the way.

A special thank you goes out to Lisa, Paul, Christine, Katie, Jess and the entire team at Rockpool. Your dedication and expertise have been invaluable in bringing this project to fruition. I am also grateful to Tamsin Holmes, whose culinary talents added depth and deliciousness to the content, and to Rob Palmer for his photographic contributions.

I am deeply appreciative of my friends, mentors, colleagues and contributors, who have offered their insights and encouragement throughout this journey. To my fellow long-haulers, your shared experiences have provided strength and solidarity. Thanks to Lizzie Williamson and Sebastian Thaw for graciously allowing me to share their stories.

To my family, your unwavering love and support have been my guiding light. Tamsin, Oscar and Tinkerbelle, you bring joy and inspiration to my life each and every day.

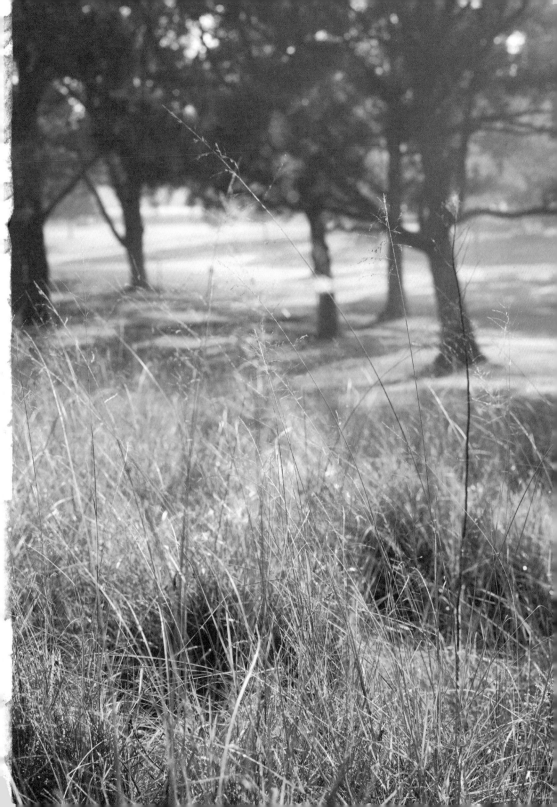

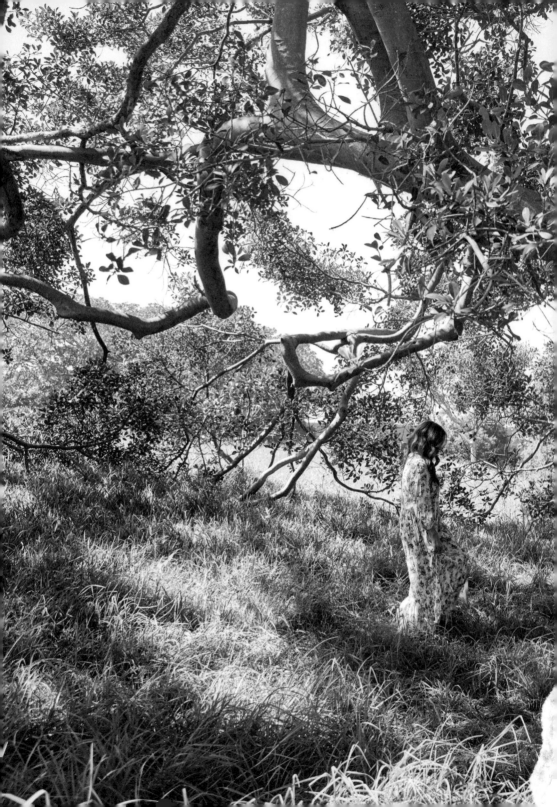